MW00830276

MATERIA MEDICA
MEXICANA

A MANUAL OF
MEXICAN MEDICINAL
HERBS

1904

British Library Cataloguing-in-Publication Data
A catalogue record for this book is available from the
British Library

A Short History of Herbalism

Herbalism ('herbology' or 'herbal medicine') is the use of plants for medicinal purposes, and the study of such use. It covers all sorts of medicinal plants, natural remedies or cures, traditional and alternative medicines. Modern medicine tends to categorise herbalism firmly as an 'alternative therapy' as its practice is not strictly based on evidence gathered using the scientific method. Modern medicine does make use of many plant-derived compounds however, as the basis for evidence-tested pharmaceutical drugs. *Phytotherapy* also works to apply modern standards of effectiveness testing to medicines derived from natural sources.

Medicinal plants have been identified and used throughout human history. Archaeological evidence indicates that the use of medicinal plants dates at least to the Paleolithic age, approximately 60,000 years ago. Written evidence of herbal remedies dates back over 5,000 years to the Sumeranians, who created long lists of useful plants. A number of ancient cultures wrote on plants and their medical uses. In ancient Egypt, herbs are mentioned in Egyptian medical papyri, depicted in tomb illustrations, or on rare occasions found in medical jars containing trace amounts of herbs. The earliest known Greek 'herbals' were those of Diocles of Carystus, written during the third century BC, and one by Krateuas from the first century BC. Only a few fragments of these works have survived intact, but from what remains scholars have noted that there is a large amount of overlap with the Egyptian herbals.

Seeds likely used for herbalism have been found in archaeological sites of Bronze Age China dating from the Shang Dynasty, and herbs were also common in the medicine of ancient India, where the principal treatment for diseases was diet. *De Materia Medica* (an encyclopaedia and pharmacopoeia of herbs and medicines), written between 50 and 70 AD by a Roman physician, Pedanius Dioscorides, is a particularly important example of such writings; focused on the diet and 'natural remedies.' The documentation of herbs and their uses was a central part of both Western and Eastern medical scholarship through to the eighteenth century, and these works played an important role in the development of the science of botany too. Dandelion for instance, was used as an effective laxative and diuretic, and as a treatment for bile or liver problems, whilst the essential oil of common thyme was (and is) utilised as a powerful antiseptic and antifungal. Before the advent of modern antibiotics, oil of thyme was additionally used to medicate bandages.

The fifteenth, sixteenth and seventeenth centuries were the great ages of herbal remedies; with many corresponding texts being published. The first 'Herbal' to be published in English was the anonymous *Grete Herball* of 1526. The two best-known herbals in English were *The Herball or General History of Plants* (1597) by John Gerard and *The English Physician Enlarged* (1653) by Nicholas Culpeper. Culpeper's blend of traditional medicine with astrology, magic and folklore was ridiculed by the physicians of his day, yet his book - like Gerard's and other herbals, enjoyed phenomenal popularity. Natural medicines gradually waned in popularity as the 1900s progressed however, and the twentieth century also saw the slow erosion of plants as the pre-eminent sources of therapeutic effects.

Despite this, today the World Health Organization (WHO) estimates that eighty percent of the population of some Asian and African countries use herbal medicine for some aspect of primary health care. Pharmaceuticals are prohibitively expensive for most of the world's inhabitants, half of which lives on less than two American dollars a day. In comparison, herbal medicines can be grown from seed or gathered from nature at little or no cost. In actual fact, many of the pharmaceuticals currently available to physicians have a long history of use as herbal remedies, including opium, aspirin, digitalis and quinine. As is evident from this incredibly short history of herbalism and natural plant remedies – it is an aspect of human medicine with an incredibly long, varied and intriguing record. With many such traditional cures still used in the present; the multifaceted uses of plants continues to surprise us. We hope the reader enjoys this book.

INTRODUCTION.

It was the intention of the National Medical Institute to prepare a catalogue of the drugs displayed at the Paris Exposition of 1900, as it was judged insufficient to make a simple inventory without giving explanations of the characters of the drugs and of their botanical classification, physiological action, therapeutic applications and posology. Our motive was to extend thus a scientific knowledge of our medicinal plants among foreigners in order that those interested might know them more intimately and thus be enabled to use them, either in commerce or for medicinal purposes. But we were not successful in finishing this catalogue in time and, therefore, it was not sent to the said Exposition.

Now, when it became necessary to make a new catalogue of drugs for the St. Louis Exposition, the former material which had been translated into French by Dr. Ricardo E. Cicero, was utilized; additional matter corrected as far as possible, new articles being inserted, and what was wanting in the French text, added. In this way what was originally intended for a simple catalogue became a work deserving the name of "Manual of Materia Medica Mexicana."

It is based upon the extensive studies published in the "Datos para la Materia Medica Mexicana," by the Mexican National Medical Institute from which I have extracted what seemed to me most important for medico-pharmaceutical application. I have also added other data, some from my own works, some from scientific works published by the personnel of the Institute, and still others from sources which I shall mention in their proper places.

I have endeavored to make of one small volume a compendium of the material as much abridged and condensed as possible, contained in the four volumes of the "Datos para la Materia Medica Mexicana," three of which are already published; one in print, the last being forthcoming. The articles are numbered consecutively; each drug sent as a sample to the St.

Louis Exposition bearing a number corresponding to that of the article in which it is described. The compendium will also serve as a catalogue, and our medical and pharmaceutical students will be able to utilize it as a hand-book to acquire a knowledge of our principal medicinal herbs for common use. This purpose would be more readily served if the student in addition to the text had a collection of small samples of Mexican drugs; which collection could readily be furnished by the druggists or by the National Institute.

Thus the knowledge and use of our medicinal herbs will be advanced among physicians themselves and the mistakes frequently made in their use will be avoided.

MEXICO, February, 1903.

Dr. FERNANDO ALTAMIRANO.

MANUAL OF MATERIA MEDICA MEXICANA.

Artemisa Mexicana.
(Compound.)

Vulgar Syn—Estafiate, Absinthe of the country; Iztauhyatl in Mexican.

Grows—In the Mexican Valley, on the riversides, and in the mountains in cool and humid climates. It also grows in many other parts of the country, San Luis Potosi, Vera Cruz, Chihuahua, etc. Its vigorous rhizoma causes it to be propagated and produced in abundance in the same place every year. It grows from 1 to 1⅓ metres in height, is suffructicose and vertical, branching, downy and very aromatic.

Parts Employed—The leaves and flowering shoots. The leaves are sessile, alternate, gray tomentose underneath, and of a dark green color above, the inferior leaves are pinnatifid and larger than the superior ones, which are trifid or undivided with margins rolled downwards; somewhat coriaceous; very aromatic and of a strong, bitter taste. The inflorescence is resiniferous, spiciform, erect, in small heads with an ovate and tomentose involucre, which is sometimes glabrous; its receptacle is naked.

The upper sides of the leaves are spotted with glands, which are located in very small depressions. The pith contains numerous portions of crystallized matter; some of these portions are brown in color, others are transparent and prismatic.

Chemical Composition—Fat, Chlorophyl, wax, essential oil, neuter resin, two acid resins, caoutchouc, a special alkaloid, tannic acid, Glycose gum, cellulose, lignin, and saline matter. The inflorescence contains santonin in the proportion of 1,24%.

Its more important elements are: the essence, and the santonin. The essence is a very fluid liquid matter, of a light green color, pleasing to the smell, and of a bitter taste, leaving on the tongue a feeling of freshness like that produced by mint. It deviates the polarized light $+147°$. It is soluble in absolute alcohol, and in alcohol at 85, in sulphuric ether, benzine and chloroform.

PHYSIOLOGICAL ACTION—The alcoholic extract is not toxic, nor does it exert any influence, either local or general. It does not produce abortion in the rabbit. It delays the action of the gastric juices in the stomach instead of accelerating their activity, as is commonly supposed. This retardation is probably due to the neutralization of the digestive acid by the alkaline salts in which the extract abounds. As a proof of this it can be observed that the acidity of the digestive juices is neutralized after adding the absinthate preparation, which was previously remarked as being strongly alkaline.

The essence paralizes all motility in the frog, leaving the sensitivity free. It begins to be poisonous at the dose of two drops, applied by subcutaneous injection; toxic effects appear forty minutes after the injection, and death occurs twelve hours later.

The absinthate essence is apparently less poisonous than the essence obtained from the foreign absinthe (Artemisia Absinthium.)

It was observed by experiments made upon the rabbit that an interveinous injection of 0,50 c.c. of foreign absinthe essence, caused the animal's death within half an hour, while the same effect was not obtained with 3 c.c. of the Mexican absinthe essence.

Casimiroa Edulis.

Ll. &. Lex. (Rutaceæ.)

SCIENTIFIC SYN—Zantoxylon Araliaceum, Turcz.

VULGAR SYN—Cochiztzapotl, Istaczapotl, in Mexican.

GROWS—In the Mexican Valley, and in almost every village on the central plateau, in the Mixtecas (State of Oaxaca), etc. It does not grow wild, but is cultivated as a fruit tree. It is produced in abundance and does not need to be carefully cultivated. It yields yearly large quantities of fruit, which are sold in abundance in the markets at a low price, ($0,50c for 100.). Its flowering season is during the months of January and Frebruary, and it fructifies from June to October. It grows 5 or 6 meters in height with a permanent and abundant foliage. The wood is used in industrial art.

PARTS EMPLOYED FOR MEDICINAL PURPOSES—More especially the seed, but the leaves and the bark can also be used.

CHARACTER OF THE DRIED SEEDS—Ovated form, arched and compressed, somewhat reniform, with two flattened surfaces, and two edges, one of which is thin and almost straight, with a funicular raphe; the other one is bent and thick. It measures from 3 to 6 centimeters in length, and from $2\frac{1}{2}$ to 3 in thickness. Episperm, of a yellowish-white color, with outlying nervation on the outer surface, smooth and brilliant on the inner surface. The kernel is very contracted, furrowed, and free, of a waxy or ligneous consistence, covered with a thin and very adherent endosperm of a reddish-brown color. The cotyledons are white inside; their sectional surfaces are farinaceous and nonpatty, odorless, and sweet to the taste, leaving afterwards a bitter taste. The dessication of the seeds is delayed by the impermeability of the episperm; and for this reason a large numebr of seeds become changed in character, if they are not carefully dried in a warm place, and frequently moved. It is preferable to keep the episperm complete.

LEAVES—The leaves of White Sapota, are oval or eliptic, from 12 to 15 centimetres in length, and from 2 to 6 in breadth, coriaceous, brilliant, glabrous, and with a large number of glanduous points on their surfaces which become more visible if examined through a transparency. These leaves are undulated with dented margins. They have no remarkable taste, nor odor.

Large quantities of these seeds can be obtained at the price of $0,50c a kilo; but only during the fructifying season (from June to October). The leaves, and the bark can be gotten at any time, but at a higher price. The bark is most difficult to obtain, because as decortication causes the death of these trees, owners prefer not to sell it.

CHEMICAL COMPOSITION OF SEEDS—Glucoside, essential oil, fixed oil, acid resin, neuter resin, acid dyeing matter, glucose, citric acid, malic acid, special acid, gum, starch, albumen, oxalate of lime, and other ovalates.

CHARACTERS OF THE GLUCOCIDE—Casimirose. Resinous appearance, soft consistence, strong yellow color; odorless, sugar-like taste, leaving afterwards a bitter taste; soluble in water and in alcohol; less soluble in chloroform. This glucocide contains nitrogen in its composition. The fruit, the leaves and the bark contain casimirose, but it is found in larger quantities in the seeds.

PHYSIOLOGICAL ACTION—The most remarkable symptoms that can be observed in the frog, under the influence of Casimiroa edulis are paralization of motility, due to disturbance in the cerebral nerve centers. The cardiac movements become feeble and slow. Death occurs, by the paralization of the heart.

Pigeons are affected by the following symptoms: Perturbation in their motility, gastro-intestinal hypersecration, somnolence, dyspnœa, and finally death by asphyxia.

In the rabbit it causes paresis, somnolence, feebleness in the reflex, paralysis of both sensibility and motility, dyspnœa, and death by asphyxia. In the dog: Paresis, somnolence, vomiting, gastro-intestinal hypersecratio, tranquil sleep, that can become comatose with large doses; paralysis of sensibility and of motility, diuresis, paralysis of the anal sphincter, hypotermia, and mydriasis.

To sum up: The most remarkable effects caused by white sapota are a quiet sleep, analogous to physiological sleep, gastro-intestinal hypersecration, peripheric vaso-dilatation, with sanguineous hypotension, analgesia, hypotermia which can reach to 6. C.G., paralyso-motor action, and death by failure of respiration.

These symptoms are due to the effect of the active principle contained in sapota.

It could be employed in medical practice as an hypnotic, analgesic, anti-convulsive, and also as an anti-thermic. But it must not be forgotten that with some patients the drug used in large doses has a depressive effect on the cardiac action, through abasement of the sanguineous tension. Small doses can also produce disturbance in the respiratory functions. With large doses this disturbance can produce thoracic paralysis.

THERAPEUTICAL USES—It has been successfully employed in hospitals and in town-practice, as an hypnotic. It produces a quiet and restoring sleep, without nightmare or disagreeable awakening, resembling greatly normal sleep.

It has been employed also in hospitals for alienated women, to calm their mental excitation, the substance being used alone or mixed with bromide of potassium or with chloral.

The physiological properties, mentioned above, have not all been corroborated in man. Clinical science has assigned to the sapota but two useful properties, hypnotic and sedative of the cerebral centres.

Communications from physicians, and from patients, have but recently afforded the knowledge that the fruit of sapota, has another useful quality, that is of relieving rheumatic pains within a few hours. The patients who were relieved ate the fruits of sapota at dinner time (at noon) and felt so much relieved during the afternoon that some of them said they were entirely cured of their disease.

POSOLOGY—The hydro-alcoholic extract of the seed, doses of 0.50 to 5 grammes as hypnotic, to be taken one hour in advance of the time in which it is desired to produce sleep. It is taken in pills, in capsules or syrup. Extracts from the leaves and from the bark also produce sleep, though they are less active. The doses from these extracts must be taken twice as often as that of the extract from the seed. The same dose can be given to children. Its narcotic effects are not as dangerous as those of opium. It is a good substitute for this drug, so dreadful when used in children.

The active principle, the Casimirose, has not yet been put to clinical use.

Chenopodium Foetidum.

Schr. (Chenopodia.)

SCIENTIFIC SYN—Chenopodium graveolens, Lag. and Roch.; Chenopodium Schraderianum, Rœm. and Schult.; Botrydium Schraderi, Spach.; Ambrina foetida, Mocq.; Chenopodium affesum, Mart and Gal.

VULGAR SYN—Epazote de zorrillo, Epazote de toro, Epazotl, in Mexican, signifying odoriferous herb.

GROWS—In the Mexican Valley, on the borders of broken lands, on riversides, on cultivated lands. It is also found in the states of Queretaro, Guanajuato, Orizaba, and in many other places. It does not grow in abundance; its regular price is 5c a kilo. Although the plant gets dry in the country, is not deprived of its odor. It has, when dry, the peculiarity of presenting numerous small masses of resinous matter. This resin is very aromatic and can be easily separated with the aid of a fine sieve and then fanned so that the finer particles blow off.

PARTS EMPLOYED—All the plant and its essence.

GENERAL CHARACTERISTICS—The plant is herbaceous, short in growth, very branchy and aromatic, the leaves are petiolate; the inferior ones are large, the superior ones very small and close to the infloresence; the infloresence is numerous and tufty, set in dicotomic clusters; the flowers are small and glandulous. These glands turn into the small masses of resin above mentioned. Its flowering season is from June to November.

CHEMICAL COMPOSITION—Essential oil, Concrete, fatty, matter, wax, chlorophyl, acid, resin, gum, sugar, chloride of ammonium, gluco-tannin, a special alkaloid, pectic matters, tartaric acid, oxalic acid, extractive matter, bi-basic phosphate of lime, and other mineral salts.

The essential oil is the most important principle. It has a yellow color; its distinctive odor is very intense; it has a piquant and bitter taste, causing a sensation of coolness on the tongue. It is very fluid, its density being 0.842; boiling point from 172 to 175 C. G. It is soluble in sulphuric ether less soluble in alcohol. It does not solidify at the temperature of 11 C. G. It is oxygenated and becomes easily resinous.

PHYSIOLOGICAL ACTION—The essence has been used in a dose of 10 drops put into different forms and injected into the circulatory system of the rabbit, without causing remarkable symptoms. A subcutaneous injection of 24 drops of essence made in the dog, does not produce general effects, though local ones occur as intense pain and septic abscesses. The injection of 1. c.c. of this essence causes neither local nor general action.

THERAPEUTICAL EXPERIMENTS—The infusion of the herb, and the essence in different forms, has been employed by the physicians of the hospital of San André, but in every case the effects produced have proven unsatisfactory.

It was for a long time regarded as an anti-helminthic, and although it has not been used for that purpose at the clinic of

San Andrés, still it can be considered as an excellent vermicide, having been so proven by the experiments made by Doctors Rodriguez and Rangel, of Coatzacoalcos. They say that the essence is largely used there to expel the helminths so common in the people who inhabit that part of the country. Its effects are much better than those of santonine.

POSOLOGY—The essence is taken in capsules containing from 10 to 20 drops, as an anti-helminthic. The alcoholic extract can be used in doses of 4 grammes a day.

Heterotheca Induloídes.

Cass. (Compound.)

SCIENTIFIC SYN—Diplocoma villosa, Don.; Doronicum mexicanum, Cerv.

VULGAR SYN—False Arnica, Arnica of the country, Aca-huatl, according to Cervantes; Cuauteteco, according to A. Herrera.

GROWS—In the Mexican Valley, on the plains, near the cultivated lands. It grows in great abundance, and herbalists supply it to pharmacists in large quantities every year, at the price of $0.20c a kilo. Its flowering season is during the months of August and September. It is also found in some other places of the central plain such as San Luis Potosi, Aguascalientes, Queretaro, Orizaba, Hidalgo, etc.

PARTS EMPLOYED—The heads (capitulum.)

GENERAL CHARACTERISTICS—When the heads are dry they have one involucre, with multiserrate, imbricate, and closed bracts; the ligules are almost entire; the akenes are oblong and the villina is red and biserrated. The akenes and the villina are very easily separated from the rest of the flower by dessication. This plant grows generally to 20 centimetres in height. It is branchy, downy and rough.

CHEMICAL COMPOSITION—Acid resin, yellow dyeing matter, gum, tannic acid, gallic acid, essential oil (traces), glycose, concrete fixed oils, peptic and albuminous matters, mineral salts. It appears that it also contains an alkaloid.

PHYSIOLOGICAL ACTION—No remarkable effects have been observed in animals.

THERAPEUTICAL EXPERIMENTS—The physicians who have employed it have not found in it any useful properties. It is used indeed as a substitute for genuine arnica and as a vulnerary in alcoholic tincture, but the physicians who have tried it at the Hospital of San Andrés, have not observed the good effects of genuine arnica.

Loeselia Coccinea.

SCIENTIFIC SYN—Hoitzia Coccinea, Cav.; Hoitzia mexicana, Lam.

VULGAR SYN—Espinoilla, chuparrosa, Herb of the Virgin, Huichichile, Huitzitzilzin, Huitzitzilxochitl, Quachichil, and Cuachichile.

GROWS—In the Mexican Valley. It is generally found in the ravines, among the rocks or under plants of fleshy fibre. It is hardy and frutescent. It grows to about one meter in height; its flowering season is from July to October. It is found in many other places, almost all over the country where it grows abundantly and wild. The price of one kilo is $0.50c.

PARTS EMPLOYED—The leaves and the stems.

GENERAL CHARACTERISTICS—The stems are rounded, hairy, sub-ligneous and of a yellowish color, abounding in marrow and with many irregularities on their surfaces, owing to abortive ramifications.

The leaves are elliptic-rhomboidal, alternate, simple, dentated, with mucronated notches, downy on both surfaces, pinnated, and with a prominent venation on the underneath, with short petaloid, pluri-cellulated hairs. The limbs are of a stronger green color on their superior surface, friable and thorny. This last quality gives to the plant the name of *Espinosilla* (spiny). The leaves are from 4 to 5 centimetres in length and from 1½ to 2 in width. This plant has no odor. It has a somewhat bitter taste, and if it is pounded and then stirred up in water it forms a consistent and remarkable white lather.

CHEMICAL COMPOSITION—Concrete fat, neuter resin soluble in rhigolene, chlorophyl, caoutchouc, essential oil (traces), yellow dyeing matter, acid resin number 1, acid resin number 2, tannic acid, an alkaloid, gum, albuminous matters, glucose, saponin, cellulose, lignin, starch, and mineral salts. (F. Villaseñor, Inst. Med. Nac. 1898.)

The presence of saponin and of a special alkaloid were detected only by the analysis. The alkaloid was called *loeselin*.

PHYSIOLOGICAL ACTION—The plant itself and its alcoholic and etherous extracts, have been tried upon animals to test the worth of the properties so generally attributed to it by common people, viz: febrifuge, its effect as a sudorific, as a diuretic, a vomi-purgative and a preservative for the hair. The experiments were made upon dogs and rabbits. It was observed from these experiments, that vomi-purgative effects always occur when the decoction or the infusion is used upon the dog. The effect is quick, sure and does not cause important intestinal alterations. The animal recovers its normal state after two or three hours. The vomit is bilious and with abundant salivation. The aqueous extract produces the same effect. The ethereous extract has the same properties in addition that of acting when used in sub-cutaneous injections. The powdered stems used in a dose of 1 gramme, provoke vomiting within five minutes without purgative effects.

Its action as a febrifuge has never been proved by experiment. The different preparations employed to lower the temperature or the artificially produced fever having been shown impotent to produce this effect.

Notwithstanding the numerous and long experiments made upon rabbits the diuretic effects were never observed to occur in these animals. As for its preservative qualities on the hair, and its sudorific properties they are still both under observation in clinical experiments. In short the physiological effects of the loeselia are, vomi-purgative with augmentation of the bilious secretions, without causing any symptoms of intoxication. The manner in which it acts on the digestive organs is still undetermined, but it will probably be found due to the saponin, which is abundant in this drug.

THERAPEUTICAL EXPERIMENTS—It has been employed against typhus and tuberculosis in a large number of cases at the hospitals of San André and Juarez, and the experiments have been unsuccessful to obtain the antithermic, diuretic, and diaphoretic properties that have been attributed to the drug by the antique physicians and by common people. The vomi-purgative effects have occurred in man while searching for the febrifuge effects of the drug, these vomi-purgative effects have occurred, but in a transitory and inconstant manner.

The clinical investigations made on the plant till now, have not been successful enough to expect useful therapeutic properties from it. The most that can be obtained from the drug, is to employ it as a succedant of the Virginian Polygala, on account of the remarkable quantity of saponin that the Lœselia contains. It could be used too, as an expectorant.

POSOLOGY—The following preparations and doses have been employed in man: Alcoholic tincture—30 grammes, as febrifuge; Aquous extract,—2 grammes Hidro-alcoholic extract,—4.50 grammes, both extracts as febrifuges and emetics. The decoction (10%) has been used in doses of 150 grammes a day.

Prunus Capuli.

Cav. (Rosaceous.)

SCIENTIFIC SYN—Cerasus capuli, Ser,; C. capuli, D. C.; Prunus serotina, Ehrhart.

VULGAR SYN—Capolin.

GROWS—In the Mexican Valley, cultivated or wild. It grows spontaneously at the foot of the mountains in cool and wet climates. It is a large tree of an agreeable appearance, which produces abundant fruit used as food; its wood is employed in carpentry and cabinet making.

The greatest number of large trees of the kind that I have seen, form a forest between Huauchinango and Tulancingo. Their flowering season is during the months of January and February, and they fructify from May to August.

PARTS EMPLOYED—The leaves and the bark.

GENERAL CHARACTERS—The leaves are lanceolate or lanceolate-oblong, serrate with callous notches, with one or many reddish glands at the apex or at the base of the petiole, the petioles are short, robust and of a reddish color, the stipules are lanceolate-accuminate, denticulate, glandulous and deciduous.

CHEMICAL COMPOSITION OF THE LEAVES—Essential oil, concrete fat, acid, resin with glycosidic functions, amygdaline, alkaloid, tannic acid, glycose, pectic principles, coffee-brown dyeing matter, chlorophyl, and salts. (Lozano, Inst. Med. Nac.). The fat is found in the proportion of 4%. The alkaloid has the aspect of a resinous, colorless, soft matter, it has a special odor, slightly soluble in water, soluble in alcohol, ether and chloroform. It gives the different reactions of alkaloids. The cyanhydric acid is not already formed in the leaves, but it is produced under the influence of maceration in water and can be separated by distillation. This is the process followed by the pharmacists to obtain the distilled water of capolin, which they use as a succedant of laurier-cerise water, this substitution has been approved by the Mexican Pharmascœpists.

CHEMICAL COMPOSITION OF THE BARK—Starch, resin, tannic acid, galic acid, fatty matter, ligneous tissue, red dyeing matter, calcium, potassium and iron salts (Proctor, U. S. Dispensatory). Mr. Proctor, obtained by distillation, cianhydric acid and an essential oil analogous to that which is extracted from bitter almonds.

Mr. Lozano of the Mexican Institute, found too, that the leaves and the bark contain amygdalin and a special alkaloid that had not been detected before. He did not find any phlorihitzin, although he made a minute investigation in barks of different ages and chosen from different parts of the tree.

PHYSIOLOGICAL ACTION—The extract of the leaves has been inert. The infusion of the bark (10%) is also inert. The essential oil extracted from the bark, has, on the contrary proved so active, that a dose of two drops has been enough to kill a cat in less than five minutes.

THERAPEUTIC EXPERIMENTS—The anti-periodic effects that people attribute to the bark, were not verified. The decoction of the bark has proved useful against diarrhœa, the distilled water of the leaves has proved a very useful anti-spasmodic, that has been thoroughly tested in the clinic of San Andrés and this distilled water can be used as a good substitute for the laurier-cerise water. It must be always kept in mind that the cianhydric acid is not produced if the disilation is made with dried leaves.

POSOLOGY—The distilled water is used in the same doses as the lauro-cerise distilled water. The decoction of the bark in the proportion of 5%, as an anti-diarrheic and as a tonic.

Peperomia Umbilicata.

Ruiz and Pav. (Pepperaseous.)

SCIENTIFIC SYN—

VULGAR SYN—Pimienta de tierra (Earth pepper).

HABITAT—It grows abundantly in the Mexican Valley, and in many other places such as, Real del Monte, Zimapan, San Luis Potosi, Oaxaca, etc., in soft and wet lands around the rocks and bushes. The gathering of the drug becomes expensive for the reason that the plant grows, widely scattered here and there in the country, so that, it is necessary to go long distances to get a good supply. This difficulty, could be overcome by cultivating the plant under suitable conditions. The price of one kilo is $0,50c.

PARTS EMPLOYED—Those used by the Indians, in substitution of the genuine pepper, are the tubercles which have the hot and pungent taste of the plant from which it has taken its name.

Argemona Mexicana.

Lin. (Papaberacecus.)

VULGAR SYN—Chicalote.

GROWS—This plant grows in the Mexican Valley and almost all over the Republic. It is specially abundant in the state of Queretaro where the seed can be more easily obtained at the price of —— a kilo.

PARTS EMPLOYED—The leaves, capsules and seed.

GENERAL CHARACTERS—This plant is from 50 to 75 centimetres in height, and has a very long, tapering root; the stem is thorny and glaucous, the leaves are simple, pinnatifid, with coarsely dentate lobes and with sharp, rigid thorns upon the venation; inflorescence solitary. The flower is white with numerous stamens; the fruit a spiny capsule, dehiscent at the apex. It contains numerous grains of a brown or blackish color, seeds are small, with a granulous spermodermis and contain a large proportion of oil. Its flowering season is from April to October. Among the general characters of this plant, it is worth noticing that when a leaf or a stem are cut off a yellow colored liquid oozes from the cut.

Chemical Composition of the Leaves—They contain morphine.

Chemical Composition of the Seed.

	Per Cent.
Oil	36.20
Water	7.40
Mineral Salts	5.60
Sugar	4.38
Gum	2.54
Caseine	.32
Albumin and gluten	13.38
Fecula	17.72
Ligneous	16.52
Loss	1.94
Total	100.00

—*Charbonnier.*

General Characters of the Oil.—It is very fluid, transparent, yellow in color with an oily taste and odor, leaving afterwards an astringent effect. It solidifies at 7 C. G., it is soluble in 5 or 6 times its volume of alcohol at 90°, it is also soluble in absolute alcohol, in petroleum ether, in sulphuric ether, in carbon disulphide and in chloroform. It is very drying, and the air makes it quickly oxidize and resinify. From several experiments made with the oil, it can be said that it contains a sour and volatile principle to which are chiefly due the emeto-catartic properties of the oil, this principle is not enduring and therefore the emeto-catartic properties of the oil, soon vanish away for the same reason.

Physiologic Action—The decoction and the extract of this plant were employed upon the dog without obtaining any effects resembling those of morphine, but it must be remarked, that these animals are little sensible to the action of the latter alkaloid. All the effects of opium were produced with the same preparations, when they were employed upon the rabbit. Man, too, is very sensitive to the action of this drug. In short, the Chicalote must be taken as a narcotic analogue of morphine. The oil extracted from the seed by means of the carbon disulphide produces its emeto-catartic effects, 2 or 3 hours after the injection. The oil obtained by expression of the seed has proved inactive.

THERAPEUTICAL EXPERIMENTS—According to the opinion of Doctors Terres, Govantes and Sosa, who have made numerous clinical observations, this drug should be useful against insomnia and to sooth the irritation of coughing. When the oil has been employed internally in doses from 30 to 45 drops it has produced such different effects that its use is not advisable.

People use the oil to varnish the skin in the same manner as is done with colodion, utilizing thus the drying properties of the oil when it is applied in a thin coating.

POSOLOGY—The extract of the capsules without the grains, the extract or the decoction of all the plant.

Of the hydro-alcoholic extract of the fruit, 2 grammes divided in 4 pills one to be taken every half an hour.

Of the fresh plant, coarsely ground 10 grammes, water 125 grammes, extract of liquoris S. Q. to make a decoction to be taken at bed time, as an hypnotic and pectoral. If the desired effect is not obtained the first formula may be used. Children who are sensitive to the opium preparations, will bear very well the action of the chicalote, and for this reason this medicine, is prescribed in cases of convulsive cough or other spasmodic affections.

Llora Sangre.

SCIENTIFIC SYN—Bocconia arborea, Watson.

VULGAR SYN—It is called Enguande, in Michoacan.

GROWS—In Uruapam, Tingambato, Michoacan and Jajalpa, (State of Morelos).

PARTS EMPLOYED—The bark and the yellowish-red juice that can be obtained by the incisions made in the tree.

CHEMICAL COMPOSITION OF THE BARK:

	Per Cent.
Water	10.000
Ashes	9.500
Fatty matter	1.320
Benzoic acid	0.056
Resin	9.364

4 Alkaloids
1 Bocconieritrin,
2 Bocconichlorin,
3 Bocconiiodin,
4 Bocconixantin,
.... 5.116

Gum	1.875
Dextrin and analogues	5.775
Free organic acids	2.430
Ligneous, red and yellow dyeing matters	44.990
Loss	9.574
Total	100.000

—*Inst. Med. Nac. M. Lozano.*

The bark, which is the part employed in medicine, depends for its value on the action of the four alkaloids mentioned above. Its industrial uses, are due to the presence of dyeing matters.

PHYSIOLOGICAL ACTION—The first preparation that was employed in investigating the physiologic action of this drug, was called *Bocconin.* It is a substance that is almost constituted by the mixture of the four alkaloids. It was found from the first experiments made on animals, that this substance produced very remarkable anæstetic effects. It was observed afterwards that when the bocconin was employed in man, there was intense pain in the place where the medicine was applied, before the anæsthesia occurred. After searching for an explanation of these two opposite symptoms produced by the drug, it was admitted that it depended on the different action exerted by the alkaloids constituting the mixture, some of them being irritant, and the others anæstetic. The different effects produced by each of these alkaloids, was found to be as follows:

1. The Bocconieritrine, soluble in sulphuric ether, was found to be less analgesic than the following alkaloids, but more irritant.

2. The Bocconichlorine, soluble in the absolute alcohol, acted as a local and general anæstetic.

3. The Bocconiiodine, soluble in water, was almost inert.

4. The Bocconixantine, soluble in the chloroform, appeared to have a doubtful action.

As we have stated above, these four substances are the constituents of the Bocconin. This substance is partly soluble in water, irritant, analgesic and toxic. The dose used on a frog was 2 centigrames, and it was sufficient to kill the animal 20 minutes after the application. A rabbit died from a dose of 3 centigrammes and a dog with that of 5 centigrammes. In short, the Bocconin exerts its principal action upon the nervous system, producing, at first, a painful symptom and afterwards local anæsthesia. As for the general anæsthesia, it appeared associated with some narcotic symptoms but without any perturbation of the intellect. At the same time a considerable dilatation of the peripheric vessels occurs, this dilatation may in some cases produce incoercible hemorrhages. The Bocconin was also employed as an occular anæstetic, and it was observed that it caused a painful irritation in the conjunctive and at the same time it produced opacity in the cornea, these effects will be an objection to the application of this medicine to man. The different symptoms produced by the bocconin, are doubtless due to the variable composition of this chemical. It could be said as a consequence of the physiological experiments made up to the present time, that the bocconin will be very useful in every case of painful surgical operations. The effects produced by the bocconin may be compared to those produced by an association of chloroform and cocaine employed in the same way.

The chlorhydrate, the acetate, or the citrate of bocconin, at doses of 1 to 3 centigrammes in hypodermic injections.

The Bocconichlorin or its chlorhydrate, at doses of 1 to 2 centigrammes. The following is a formula for subcutaneous injection:

Bocconin ....0.06 gr.
Distilled water 6.00
Citric acid ....S. Q. to dissolve.

One cubic centimetre of this solution is first injected in the place where the anæsthesia is wanted. The needle of the syringe is first deeply introduced and then the piston is gently pushed forward while retiring the syringe out of the place of the application.

It is most convenient to employ the medicine hypodermically utilizing it as a local anæstetic. It must not be used as an anæsthetic for the conjunctive, nor when there is any propension to hemorrhage, neither should it be used when the place where the medicine is to be injected is very sensible to pain. This precaution must be taken because, as we have stated before, the anæstetic effects are preceded by painful irritation.

Matarique.

(Compound.)

SCIENTIFIC SYN—*Caccalia decomposita,* A Gray; Senecio grayanus, Hemsley.

GROWS—In Mapula, state of Chihuahua and in the mountains of Santa Cruz, state of Sonora.

PARTS EMPLOYED—The root.

GENERAL CHARACTERS—The rhizoma is flattened and irregular, 3 centimetres in diameter, of a variable length, very tomentose and of a dirty-gray color, the transverse section presents a thin, gray circle belonging to the bark, in this circle is found a reddish brown resin that is most abundant in the inner portion of the bark; the medullary part is of a light greenish-yellow color and in it some resinous points can be observed The rhizoma gives off a great many adventitious roots from 10 to 15 centimetres in length and from 3 to 4 millimetres in diameter, round, furrowed along their length, friable, the breaking is almost a neat one, the transverse section presents a very thin, gray colored exterior circle (suber) that wraps another thicker circle brilliant and of a white color, there is after this another circle made by reddish-brown resinous points; this last circle is between the bark and the medullary part. It has an aromatic odor and a persistent bitter and pungent flavor.

CHEMICAL COMPOSITION OF THE ROOT—Resin, essential oil, glucoside tannic acid, and glucose. Henckel (from England), and M. Lozano found also an alkaloid, two resins and fatty matter.

PHYSIOLOGICAL ACTION—The hydro-alcoholic extract of the root has proven a paralizo-motor of the muscles and of the heart, it produces a light anæsthesia by its peripheric local action. The tincture facilitates the cicatrization of the tissues by exerting an antiseptic and protective action upon them, chiefly due to the coating that it forms when it is applied upon wounds, ulcers, etc.

THERAPEUTICAL EXPERIMENTS—These experiments were made with the tincture made in the proportion of one part of the plant to five parts of alcohol at 85.

Drs. Zuniga, Terres and Govantes, have observed that the effects produced by the *Matarique* when it has been taken as a purgative, are very variable; doses of 30 grames of the tincture, have not caused purgative effects but only have cured indigestion, and when the dose has been increased to 100 grames; choleriform accidents and cardiac troubles have occurred.

The useful effects obtained from this medicine are those which it produces when it is applied externally—*loco dolente.* It cures neuralgia and chronic rheumatic pains, and as we stated above it facilitates the cicatrization of wounds.

DOSES AND PREPARATIONS—The preparation that is more commonly used is the tincture made with one part of the root and five parts of alcohol at 85 F. M.

It has been used internally in doses from 30 to 100 grames, obtaining very variable effects.

When applied externally, as a vulnerary, it has been mixed with water in the proportion of 50% and the pure tincture as a pain-killer, in frictions—*loco dolente.*

Tlacoxiloxchitl.

SCIENTIFIC SYN—.

VULGAR SYN—Pambotano.

NATURAL HABITAT—This plant is found abundantly in warm places like Motzorongo, Tampico, as well as in temperate or rather cold ones, such as Amecameca near the Popocatepetl, in the Valley of Mexico, etc.

PARTS EMPLOYED—The root, in decoction.

CHEMICAL COMPOSITION—Tannic acid, fat, resin, a glucoside, pointed out by Bocquillon and Hercls, essential oil, waxy matters, etc. The glucoside was discovered by Dr. F. Altamirano, and he named it *Caliandrein*. This substance is solid, amorphous, whitish, translucent, brittle, hygroscopic, and inodorous. When it is taken into the mouth, it provokes there a somewhat sweet sensation at first, and afterwards dryness, and constriction of the pharynx are felt during some time. Caliandrein is very soluble in water, less soluble in alcohol and very little in ether. The solutions of Caliandrein give an abundant spume by agitation. This spume facilitates the emulsion of some substances and the extreme division of mercury by preventing, for a long time, the unification of the small globules of metal. It has some analogy with saponin.

PHYSIOLOGICAL ACTION—The ingestion of about 0, 90 centigrammes of Caliandrein, caused death in the dog, with the following symptoms: vomiting, abundant serous evacuations, general prostration and collapse that encreases up to death. There is no septicemia, for no bacteria were found in the blood. The caliandrein is eliminated by the bile and by the urine.

When it is employed hypodermically, the dose of 0, 20 centigrammes is enough to kill the animal; however, in this case, beside the symptoms already marked, there appears a purulent focus of necrosys at the injected place. The symptoms that we have remarked in the dog, are also produced in the rabbit, even in the case of applying the injection with all antiseptic precautions.

When the drug has been employed in man, it causes a strong sensation of constriction in the pharynx, dryness, cough, salivation and among the symptoms produced in the stomach, irritation that provokes nausea and vomiting. This symptom takes place with any dose above one centigramme of Caliandrein.

The concentrated decoction of the root, does not produce such an intense phenomena of constriction in the pharynx, although vomiting is produced and about twelve or fifteen hours later, intestinal pains are felt and evacuations occur.

THERAPEUTICAL EXPERIMENTS—It was very highly recommended in the treatment of intermittent fevers. However, according to the studies made in the Medical Institute, this medicine is not indicated against malaria fevers (paludism), because it is supposed that the hematozoa do not disappear from the blood under its action, and it has no influence on the intensity of the accesses.

It remains then to look for another medical application in conformity with the physiologic effects mentioned above.

Some physicians see in the Caliandrein, a local irritant that produces death in the tissues that it baths. According to this effect, it could be employed as a bactericide, to be applied like an antiseptic, in determined conditions.

Attention is specially called to the use of the root, which is employed in the preparation of Tepache*, with the purpose of retarding the acid and putrid fermentation of this drink. This is the action that this drug exerts in such a case.

As for the manner of using the drug in medicine, it consists in separating the bark from the woody part of the root, in order to administer separately the preparations of each. The bark will be specially used to obtain the astringent effects, and the woody part the Caliandrein for the purpose of provoking the irritant effects. It will be dangerous to employ this drug for infants and for persons of a delicate stomach, or affected with gastro-intestinal diseases.

DOSES AND PREPARATIONS—Coarse powder of the woody part of the root of Tlacoxiloxochitl, 20 gms; water, 1 kilo. Let it boil during one hour, sweeten this decoction and give it as a beverage. To be taken in three portions during the 24 hours.

Hydroalcoholic extract of the cortical part of the root, 4 grammes. To be put in pills or in capsules, containing 0,25 centigrammes each. Take two every hour.

VULGAR PREPARATION—It consists in putting about one part of the root in eight parts of water, and boiling until it is reduced to one third. To be taken as a beverage. There is a patent medicine, recommended against intermittent fevers, called *Pambotano,* this name has come to be a vulgar synonym of Tlacoxiloxochitl.

Yerba del Pollo.

SCIENTIFIC SYN—Commelina Palida.

VULGAR SYN—Rosilla, Matlalistic.

GROWS—In the Valley of Mexico in wet and shady places in the ravines. It is generally abundant and can be obtained at

---

(*) Tepache is a fermented drink, prepared with *piloncillo* (a special sort of impure sugar) and *pulque*, and, in some cases, with sugary juices and some other ferment.

the price of $0.15c a kilo. It is also found in some other places of the Republic.

PARTS EMPLOYED—The stems with the leaves and the flowers, for medical uses. The flowers, which are of a fine blue color, are used by the people to give a blue tint to sweets, the preparation is entirely harmless and gives good results. The juice of the fresh plant is also employed in medicine, but although it is much more active than any other preparation, its use has not been generalized on account of the difficulty of keeping the juice for any length of time.

GENERAL CHARACTERS—This plant is annual; herbaceous, with red, nodose, juicy stems; leaves, oblong-lanceolate, from 4 to 6 centimetres in length and from 1½ to 2 centimetres in width, entire margin, glabrous on both surfaces, and forming at the base a sheath that covers the stem, its venation is almost parallel; inflorescence, in short racemes, with two or three blue petals.

CHEMICAL COMPOSITION :

Acetic acid (in the juice).
Acetate of ammonia (in the extract).
Chloride of potassium.
Albuminous principle.
Vegetable albumin.
Chlorophyl.
Extractive matter.
and Cellulose.
1867. Herrera y Mendoza. Inst. Med. Nac.
Gum.
Neuter resin.
Acid resin.
Glucose.
Albumin.
A special tannic acid with the functions of galo-tannic acid.
Chlorophyl.
Acetic acid.

Rio de la Loza. Inst. Med. Nac. 1893.

PHYSIOLOGIC ACTION—This medicine produces strong contractions in the vessels of the mesentery in the frog. It contracts energetically the matrix in the dog and in the rabbit, these contractions being entirely expulsive and occurring by a mechanical effect similar to that of ergot and of zoapatle. It does not cause any contractions in the digestive tube nor in the organs where the excretions abound. It exerts an energetically constrictive action that is perhaps analogous to that produced by the Hamamelis virginica. Dr. Tousaint, has demonstrated by his experiments, that the effects produced by this drug are in no manner owing to the production of ammonia that occurs when the medicine comes in contact with the blood, as was supposed to take place by Professors Herrera y Mendoza.

It does not produce the hæmostatic effects by coagulation of the blood but by an energetically constringent action exerted upon the vessels, as has been stated above.

DOSES AND PREPARATIONS—The best preparations that may be used are the juice of the fresh plant or the paste made with the plant fresh or dry, but in the last case, care should be taken to dry the plant in the proper conditions, because as the stems and the leaves are very juicy, they are easily altered during the dessecation if it is not done with all possible care as to keep the plant in a well ventilated place, to maintain the temperature at the same degree of the atmospheric one, and to separate from the well preserved parts, those that may happen to rot, as soon as they appear, etc. The want of all these cares, gives for itself a full explanation for the inactivity of some of the preparations made with this drug.

The preparations that are more largely used in internal uses, are the decoction, the extract and the fluid extract. Being, this last, one of the best preparations made with this drug.

The properties of the drug may in some cases be entirely destroyed if it is submitted to the action of a strong heat or when the action of fire is maintained during a long time.

The dose of the dry plant when it is taken in decoction is from 5 to 20 gs. the extract may be taken in pills to the dose of 5 grammes.

Simonillo.

SCIENTIFIC SYN—Coniza filaginoides D. C., parvifolia D. C. gnaphalioides H. B. K.

VULGAR SYN—Zacachichis, zacatechichic.

PART EMPLOYED—The entire plant. It was employed by the ancient Astecs as an emetic, cholagogue and anti-dyspeptic.

GENERAL CHARACTERS OF THE DRUG—The decoction has a very bitter taste and it produces an abundant froth when it is shaken.

CHEMICAL COMPOSITION—

Concrete fat.	Pectic matter.
Acid resin.	Salts, and a
Chlorophyl.	Glucoside.—*Lennesin.*
Essential oil.	

Dr. F. Altamirano. Inst. Med. Nac. 1893.

CHARACTERS OF THE LENNESIN—It is an amorphous product of a yellow-greenish color and of a very bitter taste. It is soluble in water and in alcohol, slightly soluble in sulphuric ether and insoluble in petroleum ether, it is also very soluble in ammonia. The solutions of lennesin give a blackish-brown precipitate with the Molibdate of ammonia. The sodalye gives to lennesin an intense yellow-greenish color. Nitric acid changes it to red and muriatic and sulphuric acids to green.

PHYSIOLOGIC ACTION—The ingestion of the concentrated decoction, caused bilious vomiting in animals. When the same preparation was injected in the auricular vein of a rabbit, several peculiar symptoms took place and were ended with the general paralysis of the animal; the respiration and the cardiac pulsations were retarded, the urine became bloody and appeared of a blackish color, death occurred three hours after the injection. As it has been seen the lennesin, has energetic physiological properties, by exerting a strong action upon the blood and the bile.

THERAPEUTICAL EXPERIMENTS—Dr. Liceaga has employed the Simonillo with very good results against catarrh of the bilious vessels. It is a good agent against jaundice on account of its cholagogue properties and it prevents, too, the repetition of hepatic colics.

Doses and Preparations—The most useful preparation, is the infusion made with 5 grammes of the coarsely ground plant into 200 grammes of boiling water. The hydro-alcoholic extract can be used in doses from 2 to 5 grammes. As for the Lennesin, it can be used in doses from 10 to 40 centigrammes. The following formula is highly recommended against flatulency and constipation:

Simonillo coarsely ground .... 20 grammes
Water ....500 grammes

To be made into a decoction and applied as a clyster.

Tlalocopetate.

Scientific Syn—Coriaria atropurpurea D. C.

Vulgar Syn—Tlalocopetate by a corruption of the Mexican name *Tlalocopetlatl*, which signifies "fern of earth."

Places of Vegetation—Amecameca state of Mexico, Oaxaca, Michoacan and Chiapas. It grows abundantly on the borders of the ravines. Its common price is 10c a kilo of the fresh plant.

Parts Employed—The leaves and the fruit are used in Amecameca to poison dogs. The parts employed in the Institute to make the investigation of the properties of this plant were some branches with their leaves and others bearing their fruits and flowers.

Characters of the Plant—The entire plant is a shrub from 2 to 3 metres in height, it is very branchy from top to bottom, the branches are very long and slender, many of them leaning upon the nearest rocks or trees. The inflorescence is purple and set in long, terminal clusters from 10 to 14 centimetres in length, with large pedunculate, hermaphrodite flowers with reddish petals.

Characters of the Drug That Was Employed in the Institute—The branches that were used in the researches made upon this plant, were characterized by their cornered quadrangular and rough stems; the leaves were alternate, approximate, oblong, entire and extended, having the appearance of a fern, somewhat equilateral with projecting venation on the inferior surface, the veins being almost parallel to the length of the leaf.

CHEMICAL COMPOSITION—Fat, resin, tannic and gallic acids, mucilaginous matter, coriarin, coriamyrtin, and lime, potassium and magnesium salts.

PHYSIOLOGIC ACTION—According to the experiments made in the Institute, the Tlalocopetate had the same physiological effects of the European Coriaria, already experimented with there; such as chronic convulsions, trismus, respiratory accidents and death caused by asphyxia, besides, Dr. Toussaint observed that this medicine exerted an especial action on the heart that had not been pointed out up to date. This action consists in the slowing of the cardiac contractions and in the increase of their energy. The same effects were produced with the Coriamyrtin, that is, the pulsations of the heart were slower than in the normal state, the cavities of the heart became largely dilated and filled with blood during diastole, and emptied completely during systole.

Summing up: The cardiac energy and the arterial tension became increased and the muscular and respiratory systems were also excited.

THERAPEUTICAL EXPERIMENTS—It was not tried on man for fear of the grave toxic accidents that this drug produced in animals, although employed in small doses, and, besides, the physiological equivalent, was not established. But, judging by the physiological action of this drug, it could be tried as a cardiac tonic, succedaneous to digitalis or caffin.

Pipitzahoac.

SCIENTIFIC SYN—Perezia adnata.

VULGAR SYN—Espanta vaqueros (sowherd frightener), in Taximaroa. Cola de zorra (Foxe's tail), in the Hacinda de la Nopalena, state of Guauajuato where the stems are used by the country boys in a play that they call *cuelas* (this word is a provincialism used to denote, to go or to walk), the stems in this play are called *jaras* (arrows.)*

PLACES OF VEGETATION—The species *adnata,* almost separated from the others, is found in large abundance near Salvatierra state of Guanajuato, and between Acambaro and the lake of Cuitzeo, where large quantities of the plant can be obtained at a low price. It also grows in the Mexican Valley and is abundantly brought to the capital.

This species and some others are also found in Tenancingo and Tultenango state of Mexico, and in many other places of the Republic. It grows especially well in temperate or rather cold climates. Its flowering season is during the months of August and September.

PARTS EMPLOYED—The rhizoma and its roots, but it is preferable to use the roots without the rhizoma, since the latter contains but a small quantity of pipizoic acid and, besides, it retains a large quantity of the dissolvent employe in extracting the acid from the rhizoma. The roots, therefore, give a larger quantity of the active substance at a lower price. These roots have been used since ancient times, by the country people, to produce purgative effects.

CHARACTERS OF THE RHIZOMA AND OF ITS ROOTS—The first is hard, woody, crooked on the upper surface, bearing the supports of the new stems and scars from those that have been separated. It presents many downy portions the hairs being fine, silkly and of a yellowish color.

The roots are very thin and long (of about 20 centimetres in length and from 3 to 4 millimetres in diameter), yellowish colored, with a strong smell and a bitter taste, flexible and coriaceous; the bark of the root is easily separated from the woody part, which is flexible, fibrous and of a whitish color.

In breaking the root there appears at the broken point a yellowish circle of a resinous crystaline matter, constituted by pipizoic acid, this circle is situated between the bark and the woody part of the root. With the aid of a lens and in a strong light, the crystals can be seen very distinctly. If an identifica-

---

(*) *Cuelas:* A boys' play which consists in throwing with their hands in an oblique direction a *jara* (a long and straight stem of the Perezia) upon a smooth and level extension of ground, so as to make it to go through the longest distance. Several boys send their jaras in the same way, and the one that goes the farthest, or *cuela* the more, as the boys say, is the one that gains in the play.

tion of the pipizoic acid is desired, it will be obtained by putting in contact with the circle of crystals ammonia water or any alkaline salt, when a violet coloration will be produced. This reaction is the best one for recognizing the pipizaoac root and for detecting it among others with which it has some resemblance and that also present, in their breakage, a yellowish and resinous circle.

There are some other species of this plant, besides the species *adnata,* which also produce a purgative effect and are employed by people for this purpose, among these are the following: *P. rigida. P. dugesii. P. wrightii.* and the *P. hebeclada.*

CHEMICAL COMPOSITION OF THE ROOTS—

> Pipizoic acid.
> Acid resin.
> Essential oil.
> Tannic acid.
> A white substance that crystalizes by sublimation.
> A hard and black resin.
> Celullose.
> Galic acid.

> —*Drs. Altamirano y 'Armendariz.*

> Inst. Med. Nac. 1893.

THERAPEUTICAL EXPERIMENTS—This root is used by the Indians of Tenango as a purgative. They use it especially in cases of tabardillo, and they say that it causes perspiration and intestinal evacuations in the patient. (Dr. Ortega).

Dr. H. Carpio, obtained constant purgative effects in many cases in which he employed this drug among his patients at Hospital of San Pablo.

Dr. Terres of the Medical Institute, has tested the purgative effects of the drug on the patients of the clinic of San Andrez. He has observed also that the evacuations produced are soft or somewhat liquid without any bilious appearance, preceded by some slight colic and in some cases by vomiting. He thinks that this medicine acts on the intestinal fibres and is therefore indicated in cases in which the discharge of the intestinal tube is wanted. The purgative effects begin to be manifest two hours after the injection.

It can be employed only for the purpose of clearing the intestines in cases of constipation or as a succedaneum of aloes, over which it has the advantage of not producing or exaserbating piles. It is indicated in cases of intestinal engorgement of old people.

May it be used as a succedaneum of the Chittem bark? We think it may be employed in that manner if it is only necessary to excite the intestinal contractions without augmenting the secretions. It is an analogue to Jalapa of which it can be well used as a substitute.

DOSES AND PREPARATIONS—*Vulgar preparation*—A sweetened decoction of 4% of the fresh root, in one dose; it acts as a purgative.

The pharmaceutical preparation tried at San Andrez, was a powder of the root put in capsules at doses of 1 gramme, it acting as a purgative, certain and without unpleasant effects.

The pipizoic acid can be used in doses of 1 gramme in 10 pills; from 2 to 3 pills at bedtime in cases of constipation. They are less active than the root and they are indicated in cases of constipation, of piles and for intestinal paresia.

Panete.

SCIENTIFIC SYN—Plumbago pulchella, Boisd; Plumbago rhomboidea, Lodig. (Plumbaginaceide).

VULGAR SYN—Jiricua, Yerba del alacran (Scorpion's herb), Cola de pescado (Fish's tail), Cola de iguana (Guana's tail), Tlepatli, in Mexican signifies, fire medicine.

PLACES OF VEGETATION—In the Mexican Valley, in dry and rough lands such as the hills near the Villa de Guadalupe, la Magdalena, etc. It grows also in many other places of the Republic.

PARTS EMPLOYED—The entire plant.

CHARACTERS OF THE DRUG—The roots are rhizomatous, twisted, fascicular, from ½ to 4 centimetres in diameter, interwoven the one with the other, thick and hard; the bark of the root is dense, blackish on the outside and yellowish in the inside, it has an astringent and pungent taste; the meditulio is woody, of a reddish color and insipid. The transverse section of the root presents two zones that can be distinctly traced by the aid of a lens. The external circle constitutes the bark and has the property of producing a red coloration, in contact with the alkalies; the internal zone, is the woody part and shows a violet-red color when it is put in contact with acids.

STEMS—These are thin, round, reddish, fluted, nodulose, friable and with an abundant pith.

LEAVES—The leaves are ovate-oblong, accuminate about six centimetres in length and two in width, simple, feather-veined, amplexicaul and glabrous.

CHEMICAL COMPOSITION—

Reddish dyeing matter.	Extractive matter.
Semi-liquid fat.	Chlorophyl.
Yellowish-white resin.	Starch (traces).
Dry, black resin.	Mineral salts.

Mr. Gomez.

This plant was studied afterwards in the Medical Institute, and Dr. F. Altamirano, found the active principle of it, the *Plombagin.* It is a yellowish substance formed in spongy masses of long, fine cystals. It is soluble in cold water, but more so in boiling water from which it is deposited by cooling; soluble also in rhigolin, in alcohol and in ether and very soluble in oil. It is volatilized under ordinary temperature, and the evaporation produced provokes a strong irritation of the larynx and of the pharynx. When it is put in contact with alkalies, it gets a red-brown coloration that is changed into a yellowish one by acids. It causes discoloration and strong irritation of the skin. It gives an intense red color to the coagulated albumen of egg, this coloration penetrating deeply into the mass, and is due to the alkalinity of the albumen.

PHYSIOLOGICAL EFFECTS—The application of the leaves to the skin, causes at first, a tubefascient effect and if the action of the drug lasts during 20 or 30 minutes it will produce blistering.

The following experiment was made on a cock's comb and we observed the following alterations as a result of the application: Exfoliation of the superficial layer of epithelium, a blackish coloration, infiltration of small round cellules under the part of the epithelium that was still adherent, and also throughout the cavernous tissue. A week later, an examination was made of the place of the application and it was found that the cavernous and muscular layers had almost completely disappeared, and in their place were observed, conjunctiva and fibrous portions, strongly infiltrated with small cellules.

Gray hair and the nails, get, in contact with the drug a black coloration, more or less intense. The juice of the plant, also, has the same effect.

A solution of Plombagin in oil, causes in the skin, itching and irritation two hours after the application, and afterwards rubescence and a strong subcutaneous edema. The epithelium becomes black and the mark disappears with much difficulty. Sometimes the skin gets a permanent gray color. The subcutaneous injection of plombagin, causes a strong œdema at the place of the injection, a more or less intense black coloration of the nearest tissues, and afterwards the necrosys occurs.

This alkaloid, produces according to appearances, a sort of dry gangrene, without any general phenomena of intoxication. The necrosis is probably due to the penetrating of the plumbagin in the cellular protoplasm, for which it has a strong affinity, and makes it inadequate for fulfilling its nutritive functions.

THERAPEUTICAL EXPERIMENTS—The plumbagin may be employed for the destruction of malignant tumors, by injecting into the center of the tissue, an oily solution of plombagin. It could also be used to destroy the dental pulp, instead of arsenical and other sorts of pastes, employed by dentists. It has been successfully employed as an odontalgic, applying it directly upon the caries, taking special care to prevent its action upon the other parts of the mouth. In short, it can be considered as a revulsive, much better than iodine, because its action is more deeply manifested and the affluence of leucocytes appears in a larger peripheric zone.

DOSES AND PREPARATIONS—The alcoholic tincture of *Pañete,* made with the leaves or with the root of the plant, is active enough for the external applications.

The benzolic or the oily preparations, are very active.

Plombagin .... 0, gms 03
Sterilized oil .... 5 c. c.

For hypodermical injection.

It may be injected in small portions at several points of the tumor or in that part of the tissue to be destroyed.

Contrayerba.

SCIENTIFIC SYN—Psoralea pentaphylla, Linn.

VULGAR SYN—Contrayerba blanca o del interior. (White or inland contrayerba).

PLACES OF VEGETATION—This plant grows in the state of San Luis Potosi and still more abundantly in that of Queretaro.

PARTS EMPLOYED—The root.

GENERAL CHARACTERS OF THE DRUG—

CHEMICAL COMPOSITION OF THE ROOT—

Hygroscopic water	10.000
Mineral substances	3.750
Acid resin, essential oil, and yellow dyeing matter	3.980
Solid greasy matter, fusible at 60°.....	1.880
Acid principle, crystallizable	0.400
A special alkaloid called *Psoralin*, and Glycose	9.250
Gum	6.895
Glycose	1.440
Starch	26.500
Vegetal albumen	1.000
Cellulose and lignine	28.750
Loss	6.154
Total	100.000

—*M. Lozano y Castro. Inaugural Thesis. 1899.*

The active principle of this plant, is the alkaloid discovered by Mr. Lozano and called *Psoralin*. It can be obtained in the proportion of 9%. It crystallizes in colorless, translucent needles; it has an aromatic odor and a bitter taste; it is very soluble in hot water, soluble in alcohol at 90°, in acetic ether, in chloroform and in glycerin. When the alkaloid is subjected to the action of heat, it melts and then it is sublimated and crystallized. Treated by diluted acids, it forms crystallized salts, soluble in water.

PHYSIOLOGICAL ACTION—The powder and the fluid extract, have not produced any symptoms of intoxication, although taken in doses of 100 grammes. Vomiting, and purgative effects are the only phenomena observed in such cases. The alkaloid is toxic in a dose of 3 grammes, without provoking evacuations. The Psoralin is quickly absorbed by the stomach, or applied hypodermically, and it is, as well, quickly eliminated. It is a peripheric and pulmonic vaso-dilater. As an anti-thermic it has an action that resembles greatly that of antipyrin, but without provoking the secondary effects of the latter substance.

Dr. Toussaint has said of the physiological action of Psoralin that:

First. When the Psoralin is taken in small doses it does not cause the lowering of the normal temperature.

Second. It proves useful against the hyperthermic condition when this has been artifically provoked, and against the fever caused by toxins.

THERAPEUTICAL EXPERIMENTS—From the several observations that have been made by Drs. Huici and Terrés at the Hospital of San Andrés, by Dr. Vergara Lope at the Hospital Béistegui and by Dr. Govantes on some of the patients who come for consultation at the Medical Institute, we ascertain that this drug has a useful action in the treatment of intermittent fevers.

DOSES AND PREPARATIONS—Contrayerba root in powder, 10 grammes. To be taken in two doses; one at the beginning and the other at the end of the access.

The maceration of contrayerba in Sherry wine, may be also employed. The fluid extract is used in doses of three grammes. The crystallized psoralin, in doses of 0.10 to 0.20 centigrammes, in hypodermic injection.

Arbol del Peru.

SCIENTIFIC SYN—Schinus molle. Linn.

VULGAR SYN—Pelonquahuitl, Copalquahuitl, Pimienta de America, (American pepper).

PLACES OF VEGETATION—In the Mexican Valley and almost all through the Republic. It occurs even in very poor and saline soils.

PARTS EMPLOYED IN MEDICINE—The leaves, the fruits, the gum-resin and the essence obtained from the leaves and from the fruits.

GENERAAL CHARACTERS—*The Leaves*: Are imparipinnate (odd-pinnate) multijugulate; the leaflets are almost sessile, sharp-lanceolate, finely serrate, smooth, of a brilliant green color above and opaque underneath, the terminal leaflet being larger than the others.

The Fruit: Is small, about three millimetres in diameter, round, of a red color, when it is ripe; the epicarp is stiff and brittle; the endocarp is hard, covered with a peculiar sweet substance and contains one seed.

The gum-resin: Is a white, odorless substance, with a sour and bitter taste, it melts at 40° and forms with the water a permanent emulsion.

The essence: The essential oil is a fluid, colorless or light-yellow substance, its odor is that of the tree; it is less dense than water (D. 0.852), its boiling point is between 64° and 143° C. G., it is soluble in alcohol, in ether and in chloroform, though almost insoluble in water.

CHEMICAL COMPOSITION OF THE GUM-RESIN—

Gum	40.00
Resin	60.00
	100.00

—*M. C. Jiménez.*

CHEMICAL COMPOSITION OF THE FRUITS—

Glycose.	Leptin.
Resin.	Tannic acid.
Essential oil.	Cellulose and salts.

The fruit is the part of the tree which contains the active principles that could be employed in therapeutics.

M. C. Jiménez.

PHYSIOLOGICAL ACTION—The experiments made by Dr. Toussaint, have proved that the gum-resin causes an intense gastro-intestinal inflammation when it is taken in emulsion in water and in doses of two grammes. This inflammation is evinced by vomiting and abundant bloody evacuations; these symptoms are followed by a profound depression, weakness and frigidity. Death occurs about 24 hours after the ingestion of the drug.

It can be observed by an autopsy that the viscera are strongly congested, the stomach and the intestines are full of a liquid, black blood and the biliary vesicle is filled up.

The effects of the gum-resin are only purgative if it is employed in therapeutical doses. The essence appears to be well tolerated; it is eliminated by the kidneys and lungs.

THERAPEUTICAL EXPERIMENTS—Dr. F. Altamirano has employed successfully the essence of the Schinus molle to cure genito-urinary diseases. Mr. Bertherand has used the fruit in the form of pills as an anti-blennorrhagic; and it can be ascertained from his observations that it is a good medicine in cases of genito-urinary diseases. He thinks that the effects of this drug are much better than those of cubebs.

The emulsion of the gum-resin has been employed with success by some physicians to clean the spots of the cornea and to cure wounds.

Dr. Orvañanos, has used the gum-resin in doses of 0.60 centigrammes divided in 6 pills, as a purgative and as a modifier of the respiratory apparatus.

DOSES AND PREPARATIONS—

Leaves of Schinus molle .... 30 grammes
Water .... 500 grammes

To make a decoction for external use.

The gum-resin may be used in doses of 0.50 to 0.60 centigrammes in pills to be taken in 24 hours. A concentrated solution of it can be employed for external applications.

Essence of Schinus molle ...0.50 centigrammes.

In five capsules to be taken in 24 hours.

Yoyote.

SCIENTIFIC SYN—Thevetia Yccotli, D. C., Cerbera thevetoides, H. B. K.

VULGAR SYN—The fruit is commonly known by the name of "Codo de Fraile" (Friar's elbow.)

PLACES OF VEGETATION—This shrub grows in the hot climates of the Republic and most specially in the states of Morelos, Michoacan and Guerrero.

PARTS EMPLOYED—The seed.

CHARACTERS OF THE DRUG—

CHEMICAL COMPOSITION OF THE SEED—According to the analysis made by Prof. Herrera, the seed of yoyote contains among others the following principles:

> Vegetable caseine.
> Fixed oil, non-secative, in the proportion of 40%.
> Extractive matter
> and Thevetose. This is the toxic principle of the drug.

In the samples of the drug that have been analyzed at the Medical Institute, it has been found that the oil was in the proportion of 64%.

Prof. Warden of Calcutta, has also found the Thevetin and a yellow colored substance that he called *pseudo-indican.* The presence of this substance in the urine, will be found useful to detect the ingestion of the poison, for the reason that it has the property of producing indigo when it is put in contact with an oxydant and muriatic acid.

PHYSIOLOGICAL ACTION—Dr. Toussaint has observed that the injection of 0.05 centigrammes of the aqueous extract, under the skin of a dog, is enough to cause, within a few minutes, the following symptoms: Vomiting, intestinal evacuations, agitated breathing, progressive prostration and death; this is in some cases preceded by convulsions. The movements of the heart, become in some cases very slow and very frequent and arhythmic in others. Vomiting is provoked by central (vulvar) action, and death occurs by paralysis of the heart.

The following phenomena occur in the circulatory apparatus: Diminution of the rhythm in the cardiac contractions and augmentation of arterial pressure. The retardation in the number of the cardiac contractions is due to the exitation of the in-hivitory intra-cardiac system, as has been demonstrated by the experiments made by Dr. Toussaint. These consisted in paralyzing the system by the influence of atropin, and then an injection of yoyote is applied, having been observed in this case that no alteration took place in the number of contractions.

The arterial pressure is augmented at the beginning of the experiment and it diminishes afterwards. In one of the experiments made on a dog, the arterial pressure was augmented from 140 to 240 millimetres and came down to 0, when death occurred.

THERAPEUTICAL EXPERIMENTS—Thevetose has been employed, although with little success, as a succedaneum of digitalis. The yoyote has been employed externally as a pile ointment, and has had a well marked analgesic action.

_____

Madrono Borracho.

SCIENTIFIC SYN—Arctostaphylos arguta, Zucc.

VULGAR SYN—Madroño borracho (Drunk strawberry), Garambullo.

PLACES OF VEGETATION—It grows abundantly in the mountains of the Mexican Valley.

PARTS EMPLOYED in the Medical Institute, to make the experiments: The fruits, and the leaves.

CHARACTERS OF THE PLANTS—The leaves of madroño borracho are coriaceous, of a brilliant green color above and white underneath, glabrous, serrate, and lanceolate; the flowers are white, small, pendulous, with calyx and peduncles of a red color; the fruit (berry) is very abundant, of a dark red color, tuberculous, of the size of a chick-pea, and of a sweet and astringent taste. Its flowering season is from April to June.

Chemical Composition of the Leaves—

Vegetal wax (fusible at 33°)............. 2%
Essential oil ....
Glucoside 3%
Tannic acid 7%

> Neuter resin (soluble in petroleum ether.)
> Acid resin (soluble in alcohol.)
> Glucose.
> Pectic matters.
> Albuminous matters.
> Dextrine.
> Chlorophyl.
> Yellowish-red dyeing matter.
> Mineral salts.

M. Lozano y Castro, Inst. Med. Nac. 1900.

Chemical Composition of the Fruits—

Solid fat 0.48%
Essential oil.
Caoutchouc 0.20%
Glucoside. (The same as that found in the leaves.)
Tannic acid.
Glucose...................... ....53.00%

> Dyeing matter.
> Pectic principles.
> Oxalic acid.
> Chlorophyl.
> Mineral salts.

M. Lozano y Castro, Inst. Med. Nac. 1900.

Physiological Action—As we have stated above, the leaves and the fruits were the parts employed in these researches.

Leaves. These were employed in powder, in decoction and in petroleic, ethereous, alcoholic and aqueous extracts.

These were applied by gastric and hypodermic means on dogs, rabbits and pigeons with the following results:

The powder of the leaves, did not cause any toxic effects, but only purgative. The aquoeous extract provoked astringent effects. The doses employed were:

Petroleic extract, till .... 4 grammes
Ethereous extract, till.............. 3 grammes
Alcoholic extract, till ....

Dried Fruits: They did not exert any remarkable toxic or hypnotic action as might have been expected from the enervating properties which are attributed to them. The fresh fruit seems to be active but non-toxic. It produces in the pigeon a well marked hypnotic action in doses of 0.20 c.c., employed hypodermically.

The doses employed were very strong—100 grammes for the dogs, 25 grammes for the rabbits, and the juice of 100 grammes of the fruit (20 c.c.) for the pigeons.

THERAPEUTICAL EXPERIMENTS—It was found that it exerts a hypnotic action similar to that produced by the white zapote (Casimiroa edulis.) It does not cause any trouble to the patient, neither during sleep nor afterwards.

The fruit is more active when it is fresh and has purgative effects.

DOSES AND PREPARATIONS—Hydro-alcoholic extract of the dried fruits from 1 to 1.50 grammes.

Atanasia amarga.

SCIENTIFIC SYN—Brickelia cavanillesii, A. Gray.

VULGAR SYN—Prodigious herb, Calf's herb.

PLACES OF VEGETATION—This plant is found in great abundance in the Mexican Valley and in many other parts of the Republic.

PARTS EMPLOYED—The leaves and the flowers.

CHARACTERS OF THE DRUG—The leaves are oblanceolate, serrate and villous. The leaves of the genuine plant are easily recognized by the presence of numerous glands on their surface, these glands look like small brilliant points and are found on the inferior surface. If a microscopical examination is made of the powdered leaves, the small glandulous points are easily detected, it is also noticed that the hairs are constructed of oblique, glandular cellules with small crystals in their interior.

These characters are very useful in distinguishing the genuine *atanasia* (Brickelia cavanillesii), from the false specimens which are so numerous.

CHEMICAL COMPOSITION—This plant contains the following principles:

> Essential oil.
> Fat.
> Acid resin.
> Brickelin (Glucoside.)
> Tannic acid.
> Dyeing matter.
> Chlorophyl.
> Gum.
> Starch.
> Mineral salts.

—Francisco Carmona, Inst. Med. Nac. 1894.

Both the resin and the brickelin may be considered as the active principles of the drug. The following are the characters of these substances: The resin is soft, of a brown reddish color, soluble in alcohol at 85° as well as in the same at 100°, in sulphuric ether and in alkaline solutions. Muriatic acid gives to the resin a greenish color, sulphuric acid, a brown one which becomes black afterwards, and nitric acid produces a red color. The resin has not any glucoside functions. Brickelin is a glucoside. It crystallizes in white, silky needles, which have a slightly bitter taste. It does not contain any azote, and it is not precipitated by the reactives of the alkaloids. It is soluble in hot water, less soluble in cold water, in absolute alcohol, and in a mixture of alcohol and ether. Nitric acid gives to it a blood-red color which endures the influence of heat. Sulphuric acid and bi-chromate of potash, produce a red coloration, which passes into a greenish-black one; muriatic acid, produces a yellowish color which is made more intense under the influence of heat.

PHYSIOLOGICAL ACTION—It does not produce any general action and it is not toxic. Its action upon the gastro-intestinal apparatus, is manifested at first by a bitter taste, not disagreeable, and salivation; then there is an augmentation in the secretion of the gastric juices, and consequently the appetite and the gastric movements are both excited. It acts as well as an antiseptic by diminishing or checking the activity of the putrid fermentation of food in the stomach. It does not appear to act as a tenifugue (vermifuge.)

THERAPEUTICAL EXPERIMENTS—It has been successfully employed against indigestion, in cases of dilatation of the stomach and against dyspepsia. It could be also employed with success in those cases of diarrhœa due to atony in the secretory and motory powers of the gastro-intestinal apparatus.

DOSES AND PREPARATIONS—The decoction or the theeform infusion, must be preferred in cases of dyspepsia. The ingestion of the drug will produce more successful effects if it is taken 2 or 3 hours after meals. The same preparations must be preferred if an antiseptic purpose is in view, for the reason that the decoction or the infusion will become more perfectly mixed with the food, and the medicine will come in contact with a larger portion of the stomach.

If it is needed to obtain the effects of the medicine upon the intestines, pills of the extract are to be preferred.

The infusion must be prepared in the proportion of five grammes of the leaves for 125 grammes of water. The extract is taken in doses from 0.20 to 0.50 centigrammes in a day.

Tepozan.

SCIENTIFIC SYN—Buddleia americana, Linn.

VULGAR SYN—

PLACES OF VEGETATION—It occurs chiefly between Jalapa and the Chachalacas river, and also grows in some parts of the Mexican Valley.

GENERAL CHARACTERS—This plant is a shrub that attains a height of from 3 to 5 metres, with tetragonal tomentose branches of an ochery color. The leaves are large, from 10 to 16 centimetres in length and from 5 to 7 in width, long petiolated, tomentose, obovate or oblong, dentate, of a green color above and white underneath. The stems are knotty, with abundant and irregular ramifications and of a yellow color; the bark is very thin and, with long strips of *suber* that can be easily separated. These are very aromatic.

The roots are woody, very long, fasciculated, of a yellowish color, very aromatic and with a very thin bark.

CHEMICAL COMPOSITION—The root contains the following principles:

> Fat.
> Essential oil.
> Acid resin.
> Cinnamic acid.
> Alkaloid.
> Glucose.
> Tannic acid.
> Pectic principles.
> Dextrine.
> Mineral salts.
> —*Dr. F. Villaseñor, Inst. Med. Nac.* 1900.

The most important principles are the essential oil, the cinnamic acid and the alkaloid.

Essential Oil: This has a thick consistence and is of a greenish-yellow color; its odor is aromatic and agreeable; it has a bitter and pungent taste; its reaction is acid. It is very easily resinified.

Cinnamic Acid: Only small quantities of it are obtained.

Alkaloid: This substance is solid, amorphous, of a resinous appearance, tasteless, with a peculiar odor, insoluble in cold water, slightly soluble in hot water, very soluble in alcohol, chloroform and ether. It contains azote.

PHYSIOLOGICAL ACTION—It was attempted at first to find out if this plant could exert any diuretic action, and for this purpose it was methodically experimented with for a long time on the rabbit; the decoction of the root, the extract or the alkaloid, were all employed, either ingested or given hypodermically. And from these researches we have ascertained the following facts:

First. The root of the tepozan is not toxic.

Second. It has diuretic properties.

It provokes diuresis, vomiting and more or less abundant white evacuations, whatever may be the preparation employed or the manner by which it is applied—gastric or hypodermic. Remarkable hypnotic symptoms have also been produced. It has been tried in the following doses:

Hidroalcoholic extract—From 0.50 to 1. gramme (applied hypodermically in the pigeon.)

Alkaloid—From 0.07 to 0.28 centigrammes (applied hypodermically in the pigeon.)

Hidroalcoholic extract—From 4. to 18. grammes (ingested in the dog.)

THERAPEUTICAL EXPERIMENTS—We have had occasion to prove the diuretic and hypnotic properties of this drug. It has been tried successfully for this purpose at the Hospital of San Andrés and been found also that tepozan causes analgesic effects. The decoction of the root, the extract, and the alkaloid, were employed in these experiments.

DOSES AND PREPARATIONS—Alkaloid 0.02 centigrammes. Hidroalcoholic extract, 10 grammes.

Hierba del Zorrillo.

SCIENTIFIC SYN—Croton dioicus, Cav.

VULGAR SYN—Yepacihuitl.

PLACES OF VEGETATION—It grows abundantly in the Mexican Valley, Puebla, etc. It flowering season is from August to September.

PARTS EMPLOYED—All the plant.

GENERAL CHARACTERS—

CHEMICAL COMPOSITION—The stems and the fresh leaves contain :

> Essential oil.
> Volatile oily acid.
> Acid resin.
> Neuter resin.
> Bitter principles.
> Wax.
> Chlorophyl.
> Tannic acid.
> Glucose.
> Gum.
> Pectic principles.
> Albuminous principles.
> Non determined organic acid.
> Cellulose.
> Water.
> Mineral salts.

The dried root contains the same substances with the exception of the chlorophyll and the essential oil. The dried seed contains :

> Water.
> Caoutchouc.
> Wax.
> Oily fixed acid.
> Solid fat.
> Liquid fat.
> Neuter resin.
> Acid resin.
> Bitter principles.
> Chlorophyl.
> Sugar.
> Gum.
> Albuminous matters.
> Cellulose.
> Mineral salts.

—*Dr. F. Villaseñor. Inst. Med. Nac.* 1900.

The essential oil is very fluid, of a yellow-greenish color, it has a piquant odor which resembles that of the fresh plant, and is pungent to the taste. It can be distilled between 130° and

135°. It has a density of 0.89. When brought in contact with the air it becomes less fluid and is transformed into a solid, soft mass of a dark color, which becomes black in time.

The fixed oil is of a yellowish color, transparent, when it does not contain solid fat; insoluble in water and absolute alcohol, soluble in common ether and in petroleum ether.

PHYSIOLOGICAL ACTION—The powder and the decoction of the root, have provoked vomiting. The stems and the leaves, have produced the same effects, but care must be taken to separate the tops of the stems which bear the fruit with the seed, because drastic vomi-purgative effects will occur which may, in some cases, provoke intestinal hemorrhages.

The hidroalcoholic extract of these parts of the plant has always and almost exclusively provoked emetic effects when it has been ingested. It has not produced any effect when applied by hypodermical injection. The oil of the seed is an energetic drastic purgative.

THERAPEUTICAL EXPERIMENTS—This plant has been successfully employed as a purgative at the Hospital of San Andrés. The powdered root has produced drastic purgative effects, or only slight evacuations, according to the dose employed in each case. The effects take place two or three hours after the ingestion.

The ground seed, two or three in number, have been given in capsules and purgative effects have occurred after two hours of the ingestion, with intestinal colic.

The intestinal injection made with the decoction of the leaves, has produced purgative effects analogous to those of senna leaves.

DOSES AND PREPARATIONS—Powder of the root, 1 gramme as a purgative, 0.30 centigrammes as a laxative. Decoction of the leaves 5% as a laxative.

Tatalencho.

SCIENTIFIC SYN—Gymnosperma multiflorum, D. C.

VULGAR SYN—Pegajosa, Jarilla, Escobilla.

PLACES OF VEGETATION—It grows in the Mexican Valley and in many other parts of the Republic.

PARTS EMPLOYED—The flowering submits.

GENERAL CHARACTERS OF THE PLANT—The leaves are brilliant and glutinous, their surface being covered with a thick coating of resinous matter, they do not have any remarkable odor; they are alternate, lineal, acute, entire, from 5 to 8 centimetres in length and from ½ to 1 centimetre in width. The flowers are of a yellow color and set in close corymbs.

CHEMICAL COMPOSITION—(of the leaves, the flowers and the stems) :

> Essential oil.
> Wax.
> Chlorophyl.
> Acid resin.
> Neuter resin.
> Not determined organic acid.
> Gallic acid. (?)
> Dyeing matter.
> Glucosidic matter.
> Sugar.
> Albumen.
> Gum.
> Pectic principles.
> Mineral salts.

The essential oil is obtained in the proportion of 0.77%. It is fluid, colorless, with a peculiar smell and with a sour and pungent taste. It is insoluble in water, soluble in alcohol, in sulphuric ether and in petroleum ether. It is less dense than water. Its boiling point is between 140° and 150°.

PHYSIOLOGICAL ACTION—Experiments were made with the essential oil and it was observed that it is quickly absorbed by the subcutaneous tissues. It excites, at first, the motory power of the medullar centers, but it prevents, at the same time, the functions in the extremities of the sensitive nerves of the skin and also the exitability of the muscular fibres. It causes death by paralysis of the cerebral respiratory centers.

The physiological action of the hidroalcoholic extract and that of the glucoside were also studied. The first substance produced in the pigeon, paralysis of movement, the dilatation of the pupil and somnolence. The temperature of the body came down to 3° C. G., and death occurred three hours after the application of 1 gramme of the extract by hypodermical injection. The glucoside appeared to be inactive.

THERAPEUTICAL EXPERIMENTS—Different preparations of this plant were employed at the Hospital of San Andrés, with the purpose of comprobating the therapeutical effects that have been generally attributed to it, such as vulnerary, analgesic and anti-diarrhœic.

The following are the observations obtained from these experiments: The tincture was found useful in facilitating the cicatrization of ulcer. The decoction was employed as an analgesic in some cases of muscular rheumatism, and it produced some relief. The same good effects were obtained with the hidroalcoholic extract.

The tincture proved successful when applied in friction for rheumatical or articular pains.

The decoction of tatalencho was found to be very useful as an anti-diarrhœic employed in the proportion of 6 to 10%.

DOSES AND PREPARATIONS—Infusion or decoction of the plant, in the proportion of 10%.

Hidroalcoholic extract, from 0.10 centigrammes up to 1 gramme *pro die*, as anti-diarrhœic from 0.50 up to 2.50 *pro die* as analgesic.

The tincture is applied *loco dolente*.

———

Tumba vaqueros.

SCIENTIFIC SYN—Ipomea stans, Cav.

VULGAR SYN—Tlaxcapan, Pegajosa, Espanta lobos, Limpia tunas, Tanibata, Campanula.

PLACES OF VEGETATION—It is very abundant in the state of Hidalgo, but is also commonly found in many other parts of the Mexican Valley, in dry and hard soils in cold climates.

PARTS EMPLOYED—The rhizoma.

GENERAL CHARACTERS—The tumba vaqueros is a vigorous plant, with a big rhizoma and numerous small branching stems. Its flowering season is during the months of July and August.

CHEMICAL COMPOSITION OF THE RHIZOMA—

Solid fat.
Essential oil.
Caoutchouc.
Tannic acid.
Acid resin.
Cathechine.
Glucoside.
Pectic principles.
Mucilage.
Extractive matters.
Albuminous matter.
Starch.
Lignious matter.
Cellulose.
Alumine.
Potash.
Soda.
Lime.
Magnesia.
Iron.
Sulphuric acid.
Carbonic acid.
Silicic acid.
Phosphoric acid.
and Muriatic acid.

The glucoside is the most important principle.

PHYSIOLOGICAL ACTION—This plant has not exerted any special action on animals. It has been given internally and in subcutaneous injections without producing any toxic effects nor purgative action on the intestines.

THERAPEUTICAL EXPERIMENTS—It has been commonly employed by people as a purgative and to cure epilepsy and hysteria. But the experiments made at the hospital have not had any success in such cases. However, we have comprovated the purgative effects of the plant on those patients who had taken the medicine two or three times. The evacuations are soft and accompanied with some tenesmus, and it was observed that persons who were affected by constipation experienced relief after using the medicine.

We have also observed that to obtain these effects it was necessary to choose those rhizomas that were fresh, some of them being changed by age to merely fibro-lignious matter which does not contain any resin, while others present an abundant exudation of resin on their surfaces, the latter are the only ones that have exerted any action. It is also important to remember that the Indians do not employ any part but the fresh root, and this in large doses (100 gm). These considerations are sufficient to explain the want of success with this plant as a purgative, that has been observed at the hospital, where only the dried root has been experimented with. As for the anti-epileptic and anti-hysteric action of the drug it has not been officially comprovated, but we have to remark that Dr. Sosa and other physicians who have experimented with this medicine upon their patients have had occasion to observe that it diminishes the intensity and the frequency of hysteric convulsions and that it modifies the psychic character of neurotics. Does it exert, in such cases, a direct action upon the central nervous system, or is this action indirectly exerted by means of the special effects produced on the gastro-intestinal apparatus?

DOSES AND PREPARATIONS—The decoction of the root, in the proportion of 40 or 50 grammes to 200 grammes of water is commonly recommended to be taken every day for epilepsy and hysteria. The fluid extract of the root is a good preparation. It is given in doses from 10 to 50 grammes.

The alcoholic tincture, which contains larger quantities of resin, is given in doses of 2 to 10 grammes in a day.

Chichicamole.

SCIENTIFIC SYN—Microsechium helleri, Cogn.

VULGAR SYN—

PLACES OF VEGETATION—This plant grows abundantly in the Mexican Valley, Toluca, Real del Monte, etc.

PARTS EMPLOYED—The root.

GENERAL CHARACTERS OF THE DRUG—It is a large rhizoma of about 50 centimetres in length and 6 to 8 in diameter, tapering, of a yellowish white color, odorless, bitter to taste and juicy. The transverse section presents many concentric circles which are obscure and irregular. Shaking a small portion of the root in water, it produces a profuse foam which is due to the large proportion of saponin that it contains.

CHEMICAL COMPOSITION—The rhizoma of the chichicamole contains:

> Liquid fat.
> Acid resin.
> Neuter resin.
> Saponin.
> Glucose.
> Gum.
> Dextrin.
> Starch.
> Mineral salts.

The most important principle is the saponin, it is found in a strong proportion and it is what makes the chichicamole very useful in washing linen. It can be obtained at a low price.

PHYSIOLOGICAL ACTION—The experiments made on animals, showed that this drug is very active and that its toxic effects are sufficient to produce death. The following conclusions were established after many experiments:

First. The decoction, in injection, is vomi-purgative and sialogogue.

Second. In injection it produces a hemorrhagic gastro-enteritis.

Third. The alcoholic extract is emeto-cathartic, cholagogue, tenifugue, diuretic and somewhat hypnotic.

Fourth. The greasy matter and the etherous extract have been shown to be inactive.

Fifth. The intoxication is characterized by the following symptoms: The number of the respirations is augmented at first as well as the energy of the cardiac contractions, these symptoms are accompanied by the vaso-constriction of the capillaries. There is loss of movement and of sensibility, muscular paralysis and death occurs by paralysis of respiration.

Sixth. The most active preparation is the alcoholic extract. 0.01 centigramme is enough to kill a frog, 0.05 for a rabbit and 1 gramme for a dog.

THERAPEUTICAL EXPERIMENTS—The importance of the therapeutical experiments, made at the Hospital of San Andrés, corresponds to the activity of the plant as has been shown by physiological experimentation. The cathartic action of the chichicamole, can be considered very serviceable in constipation, in cases in which some other purgatives have not proved successful. The patients who have taken it have suffered from nausea and intestinal colic. These effects were produced by powder made from the root and still more by the alcoholic extract. The tincture did not produce these effects. It was found, too, that the chichicamole, is a powerful diuretic for the cardiac, diminishing the number of pulsation and increasing the arterial tension.

DOSES AND PREPARATIONS—Powder of chichicamole, 2 grammes as a cathartic. Hidroalcoholic extract from 0.10 to 1.40 as a cathartic and from 0.30 to 0.40 as a diuretic.

Canagria.

SCIENTIFIC SYN—Rumex hymenosepalus, Torrey.

VULGAR SYN—Canaigre, Cañaigre, Cañagria,

PLACES OF VEGETATION—This plant is found abundantly over a large area in the states of Chihuahua and Coahuila. It is also found in the United States in California, Texas and Nuevo México, and can be cultivated in the Mexican Valley.

PARTS EMPLOYED—The root.

CHARACTERS OF THE DRUG—It is a tuberous root from 7 to 15 centimetres in length and from 3 to 6 in diameter, its surface is of a brown color. It has a characteristic odor and an astringent taste. It presents on its surface some sections of a reddish color, and the medullar rays are well marked, many of them are hollowed in their centers.

The microscopical examination of the powder, has shown—as an especial character of this drug—numerous small grains of starch, the polygonal cellules containing yellow masses of tannic and chrysophanic acids. These substances are characterized by the perchloride of iron, which gives a dark green coloration in contact with tannic acid, and potash reveals the chrysophanic acid by the intense red color which it produces in contact with it.

Crystals of oxalate of lime are also found in abundance.

CHEMICAL COMPOSITION—The root of Canagria contains:

Chrysophanic acid 0.90%
Gallic acid 7.00%
Tannic acid.
Gum.
Starch.
Pectic matters.
Albumine.
Mineral salts.
Water 51.00%

The composition of the Canagria varies according to the time of collection and according to the manner in which the root has been dried. It is easily altered by dampness which diminishes the quantity of tannin.

PHYSIOLOGICAL ACTION—The researches were made with the view of finding out if this drug could produce any purgative effects due to the chrysophanic acid that it contains. From numerous experiments made on animals we have concluded that it is neither toxic nor purgative, although employed at doses of 20 grammes of the powder, 22 grammes of the aqueous extract, and 1.50 of the alcoholic extract.

THERAPEUTICAL EXPERIMENTS—It has been observed that in cases of diarrhœa, the Canagria has augmented it. This is doubtless owing to the presence of the chrysophanic acid.

When it has been deprived of the chrysophanic acid by means of ether, it has checked diarrhœa of an alcoholic or tuberculous origin.

DOSES AND PREPARATIONS—Powder of the root of Canagria, from 1 to 5 grammes in a day. Aqueous extract from 1 to 2 grammes in a day.

Sangre de Toro.

SCIENTIFIC SYN—Spigelia longiflora, Mart. et Gal.

VULGAR SYN—Yerba del burro (Donkey's herb.)

PLACES OF VEGETATION—It is almost exclusively found in Real del Monte, state of Hidalgo.

PARTS EMPLOYED—All the plant.

GENERAL CHARACTERS—It is an herbaceous and perennial plant, with flowers of a fine red color. The leaves are opposite, rugose and glabrous; the stem is erect and its rhizoma is definite.

CHEMICAL COMPOSITION—

Essential oil.	Lignine.
Fat.	Potash.
Resin, soluble in ether.	Soda.
Resin, insoluble in ether.	Lime.
Tannic acid.	Magnesia.
Glucose.	Alumine.
Gum.	Iron.
Starch.	Carbonic acid.
Spigelin. (alkaloid).	Sulphuric acid.
Extractive matter.	Phosphoric acid.
Cellulose.	Muriatic acid.

—*M. Cordero, Inst. Med. Nac.* 1894.

The alkaloid is an oily substance of a yellowish color, odor *sui generis,* bitter, volatile, soluble in water, ether and alcohol. It forms deliquescent salts with oxalic and with muriatic acids.

PHYSIOLOGICAL ACTION—This plant has been shown to have very active poisonous properties. Small doses of the fresh plant have killed dogs, rabbits, pigeons, etc. They have presented the following symptoms: Paresia of the limbs, more especially of the hind ones, afterwards repeated contractions occur, which become generalized by degrees till the animal can not stand; waste of strength continues until the animal sinks into profound somnolence. The cardiac contractions which were at first much accelerated, become more and more feeble till they cease. Death occurs when the paralysis of the respiration and convulsions of asphyxia appear.

The symptoms of intoxication produced by spigelin, resemble in many respects, those produced by strychnine. Death generally occurs by asphyxia. According to Dr. Toussaint, the action of the spigelin is manifested above all, upon the central nervous system, and probably upon the spinal medulla and the rachidian bulb.

THERAPEUTICAL EXPERIMENTS—No therapeutical experimentation have been made until recently on account of the scarcity of this plant.

Ahuehuete.

SCIENTIFIC SYN—Taxodium mucronatum, Ten.

VULGAR SYN—Savino, Ahuehuetl, in Mexican language, Cpres de Moctezuma.

PLACES OF VEGETATION—It grows abundantly in many parts of the Republic.

PARTS EMPLOYED—The wood, from which is prepared the Tar of Ahuehuete, also the bark, leaves and fruit.

GENERAL CHARACTERS—Old bark appears under three different aspects; one has the form of plates or filamentous masses, which hang off from the trees in long strips; others appear in the form of logs hard and compact, of a brown color, or light, soft and of a fibrous and very irregular structure; the latter have the form of plane, fibrous and thin plates. The wood presents a different aspect according to the age of the tree. The wood of young stems is of a yellowish white color, and has not any special taste or odor. It is fibrous, lignious and soft. That of old stems is yellowish, light, soft and also without taste or smell.

Leaves. Alternate, distichous, lineal, from 5 to 15 centimetres in length, entire, a little curved, sessile, single-veined, and some of them are terminated by a mucronated, non-rigid point. They do not present any resinous exudation, but have an acid, aromatic and astringent taste, and their odor is soft and very agreeable, resembling that of fruit.

Fruits. These are of a green color, their surface covered with obtuse yellowish points corresponding to bracts which become lignified in the cone when ripe. When the fruits are not yet ripe they have a spheroid form and their size varies from that of a pea to that of a hazel nut. At the base of the peduncle, a resinous and very transparent exudation is found which possesses a strong odor. This resinous matter is also found in abundance in the fruit and can be observed by making a transverse or longitudinal section of it. This substance has the appearance of terebinthine and its odor is very agreeable.

The fruit has a very astringent and aromatic taste, but is not bitter. This is the part of the plant which contains the resin and the essential oil in the largest proportion, so that they ought to be preferred when these substances are to be extracted. The fruits are produced in great numbers every year, so many that thousands of them are not utilized at all. As the fruit and the leaves drop from the tree they could be advantageously employed in the preparation of tar and essence. The leaves are neither aromatic nor medicinally active and therefore they can not be used as a succedaneum of the genuine savin (Juniper).

CHEMICAL COMPOSITION—The leaves contain:

> Solid fat.
> Essential oil.
> Acid resin, soluble in ether.
> Acid resin, soluble in alcohol.
> Caoutchouc.
> Tannic acid.
> Alkaloid.
> Glucose.
> Pectic principles.
> Chlorophyl.
> Mineral salts.

The essential oil is of a viscous consistence, and of a reddish yellow color. Its odor is very soft and agreeable.

It oxydizes in contact with air, becoming of a thick consistence and is transformed into an acid resin. The leaves contain but very small quantities of the essence.

Fruits. In them are found the following principles:

Essential oil, density 0.825. Boiling point 130° C.
Resin, soluble in alcohol and in ether.
Mineral salts.
Tar.

One hundred and sixty-eight grammes of old, dried bark have produced, by the Aztec method of dry distillation:

Charcoal left in the apparatus.... 60 grammes.
Tar, liquid part 5   "
id id solid 2   "
Loss 101   "

The tar is produced in the proportion of 4%
The residual charcoal 36%
The water and volatile products 60%

The product obtained by distillation of the wood in a closed glass, presents the following characters: A thick, transparent liquid of a reddish brown color, with an aromatic odor and a sour and pungent flavor with a bitter after taste. Density 1147 at 15° C., and very acid reaction. It contains in 100 parts:

Acidulated water 18
Light oil (D. 1038) 9
Heavy oil (D. 1048) 40
Residues 33

PHYSIOLOGICAL ACTION—The leaves and the essence were the parts experimented on dogs, pigeons and frogs. The ingestion of the leaves in the dog did not provoke any irritant effects in the intestinal tube nor any symptoms of intoxication. On the contrary the leaves of the genuine savin have produced these conditions resulting in the death of the animals.

Several experiments were made for ascertaining if the leaves of ahuehuete could exert any special action on the matrix, but they proved to be inactive. The essence was experimented with on frogs and pigeons. It exerted a toxic action which was specially marked in the paralysis of the motor nerves of the frog and by the enervating effects produced on the pigeons.

As for the tar, it was observed that it caused anæsthesia of the buccal mucose, this symptom lasting for an hour.

THERAPEUTICAL EXPERIMENTS—The tar was experimented with producing favorable results in some cases of tuberculous diarrhœa. It was also found that it produced a strong rectal tenesmus in women. It did not prove so successful in the treatment of bronchitis.

DOSES AND PREPARATIONS—Tar of ahuehuete from 0.50 to 5 grammes in a day, in gelatine capsules.

Te de milpa.

SCIENTIFIC SYN—Bidens tetragona, D. C. Bidens leucantha, Willd.

VULGAR SYN—Aceitilla.

PLACES OF VEGETATION—It is very abundant in the cultivated land of the Mexican Valley.

PARTS EMPLOYED—All the plant.

GENERAL CHARACTERS—*Leaves*: These are lanceolate, the inferior ones serrate, and the superior ones entire, the bases are connate, and they have a glabrous surface and a soft, aromatic odor. Their taste is slightly bitter (F.M.)

Stems: These are four-angled, herbaceous and by a transverse section the four corners and the pith can be distinctly observed.

Flowers: They are almost odorless and of a yellow color.

CHEMICAL COMPOSITION—

> Fat.
> Essential oil.
> Nitrogenized matter, resembling cascine.
> Reddish-yellow dyeing matter.
> Green matter.
> *—Prof. Mendoza.*

There was not found any alkaloid nor other substance to render this plant a succedaneum of the China thee.

PHYSIOLOGICAL ACTION—It is not toxic nor has it exerted any remarkable symptoms of any kind in animals.

THERAPEUTICAL EXPERIMENTS—It has not any therapeutical applications, and has only been employed in alimentation as a theirform infusion.

Salvia de bolita.

SCIENTIFIC SYN—Buddleia perfoliata, H. B. K.

VULGAR SYN—Salvia real de México.

PLACES OF VEGETATION—It is found in Chalco, Texcoco and in many other parts of the Republic.

PARTS EMPLOYED—All the plant.

GENERAL CHARACTERS OF THE PLANT—Tetragonal branches covered with an abundant ochreous tomentose pubescence. Leaves opposite, simple, sessile, dentate, oblong-lanceolate, from 3 to 5 centimetres in length and of about 1½ centimetres in width, covered with an abundant puberscence like the stems, very aromatic and with a slightly bitter taste.

The inflorescense is glomerated, one in every axil of the flower stems with peduncles of about 1½ centimetres in length. The size of these little balls is that of a common chick-pea, they are covered with wooly hairs and are of an ochreous color.

CHEMICAL COMPOSITION—The plant contains the following principles:

Essential oil.	Chlorophyl.
Wax.	Albumin.
Fat.	Glucose.
Caoutchouc.	Tannic acid.
Acid resin.	Galic acid.
Neuter resin.	Mineral salts.
Mucilage.	

The essential oil is less dense than water, and has a yellow color and a sweet-bitter taste. It is soluble in sulphuric ether, chlorophorin and in alcohol.

PHYSIOLOGICAL ACTION—In the many experiments that have been made on animals, we could not observe any especial action of this drug.

THERAPEUTICAL EXPERIMENTS—It has been tried in abundance at hospitals and all the physicians who have employed it, have found that the tincture of *Buddleia perfoliata,* exerts a constant anhydrotic action which is efficacious and almost superior to that of the sulphate of atropin. It has been successfully employed against the perspirations of phthisis. It does not cause any trouble so that it may be used during a long time.

DOSES AND PREPARATIONS—Alcoholic tincture (20%), from 40 to 60 drops in the night some time before the perspiration begins.

Picosa.

SCIENTIFIC SYN—Croton ciliato glandulosus, Ort.

VULGAR SYN—Enchiladora, Dominiquillo, Soliman, Hierba de la cruz.

PLACES OF VEGETATION—Queretaro, Oaxaca, Chapala, Zimapan, Vera-Cruz y Tampico.

PARTS EMPLOYED—All the plant.

GENERAL CHARACTERS—The stem is round, almost shaggy and with stellate hairs; leaves ovate-lanceolate, pubescent, especially on the inferior surface, the margin of the leaves presents a great number of pedicular, piriform, small glands of a yellow color; the stipules consist of two small tufts of glands like those of the leaves; the infloressenses are set in small clusters with the female flowers at the base; the fruit is spheroid, shaggy, trilocular, tricospermous and has a pungent taste.

Liquid fat, soluble in alcohol.
Essential oil.
Caoutchouc.
Especial organic acid.
Acid resin, soluble in ether.
Acid resin, soluble in alcohol.
Glucose.
Brown-yellowish dyeing matter.
Chlorophyl.
Pectic principles.
Albumin.
Mineral salts.

PHYSIOLOGICAL ACTION—The studies of the *Picosa* are not yet concluded, we can therefore only state that the employment of a preparation made of the flowering shoots of this plant, has produced purgative action. It has also been found that it is a good antithermic.

THERAPEUTICAL EXPERIMENTS—It has been unsuccessfully employed at the Hosiptal of San Andrés, against paludism. The destruction of hematozoa has not been attested by the microscope, after the ingestion of the drug; but it was found that the temperature decreased in many cases.

DOSES AND PREPARATIONS—Decoction of Picosa 20%; from 100 to 140 grammes in a day.

Fluid extract of Picosa: 20 grammes in a day.

Chilcuam.

SCIENTIFIC SYN—Erigeron affinis, D. C.

The root of this plant is used to provoke salivation by chewing it; it is also employed against tooth-ache and in alimentation as a substitute for pepper.

It grows in the state of Queretaro, district of Toliman, San Luis Potosi and in some other places.

CHARACTERS OF THE DRUG—It is an almost globular short rhizoma, with numerous thin roots about 20 centimetres or more in length, slightly aromatic and with a piquant taste resembling that of the pellitory and which excite an abundant salivation.

Its physiologic and therapeutic effects have not been studied until recently.

Palo del Muerto.

SCIENTIFIC SYN—Ipomea murucoides, Ipomea arborea.

VULGAR SYN—Casahuate, Palo bobo, Palo del muerto.

PLACES OF VEGETATION—This tree abounds in hot and dry climates such as that of Morelos, Queretaro, etc.

PARTS EMPLOYED—Different parts of the plant were employed in the physiological experiments made at the Institute.

CHARACTERS OF THE DRUG—The stems are lignious, light, thick, of a green or gray color, united with a thin bark. The wood is characterized by very numerous concentric circles. The bark is friable and resinous, that of the young stems producing a large quantity of a milky juice which concentrates into drops of a brownish color with an aromatic odor resembling that of an old banana; it dries in contact with the air.

CHEMICAL COMPOSITION—The stems contain:

> Chlorophyl.
> Fat, in small proportion.
> Caoutchouc.
> Vegetal wax.
> Acid resin.
> Tannic acid.
> Alkaloid.
> Yellow dyeing matter.
> Chloride of ammonium.
> Glucose.
> Bitartrate of potasse.
> Gum.
> Albumin.
> Cellulose.
> Lignious matter.
> Mineral salts.

The alkaloid has a resinous appearance, a yellow color, and a very bitter taste. It is lightly soluble in cold water, more soluble in hot water, entirely soluble in alcohol, ether and chlorophorm. It is not immediately precipitated by ammonia but it gets a blue colored fluorescence.

PHYSIOLOGICAL ACTION.—A great many experiments have been made with the different parts of this plant, in order to obtain a knowledge of its toxic properties but the existence of these was not established in a definite manner until recently. The grains have in some cases produced light motor troubles. The purgative action, which is a property of the convolulaceæ, is not remarkable in this plant.

The studies of this plant were, up to the present time, prosecuted with a view to reach an exact idea concerning its toxic effects, should there prove to be any.

THERAPEUTICAL EXPERIMENTS—It has been unsuccessfully tried against the paralysis produced by cerebral hemorrhages and by arterio-sclerosis in many patients at the Hospital of San Andrés.

DOSES AND PREPARATIONS—The alcoholic tincture of this plant is employed for external applications.

The fluid extract is used in doses of 5 grammes, till 20 grammes in a day.

Cicutilla.

SCIENTIFIC SYN—Parthenium hysterophorus, L.

VULGAR SYN—Confitillo, Hierba amarga.

PLACES OF VEGETATION—It grows in the Mexican Valley and in many other localities.

PARTS EMPLOYED—The entire plant.

GENERAL CHARACTERS OF THE PLANT—It is an herbaceous and very branchy plant. The stems are striated, the leaves are large and the inflorescence tufted in glomerular bunches and of a white color.

CHEMICAL COMPOSITION—The results of the analysis prosecuted at the Institute are not yet known.

PHYSIOLOGICAL ACTION—Although it has been given to many animals under different circumstances, it has not been found toxic nor has it exerted any remarkable effects of any kind.

THERAPEUTICAL EXPERIMENTS—As we have not obtained any indication from the experiments made with this plant, it has not been employed in therapeutics.

Congora or Mazorquilla.

SCIENTIFIC SYN—Phytolacca octandra, Linn.
VULGAR SYN—Yamole, Jabonera, Poke Ing.

PLACES OF VEGETATION—It is commonly found in the Mexican Valley and in many other parts of the Republic.

PARTS EMPLOYED—The root.

GENERAL CHARACTERS—The root is tapering and very large, being in some cases one meter in length. It has a dark color is odorless and of a slightly bitter-sweet taste. It can be observed by a transverse section of the root, that it is constituted of a large number of concentric, very regular, thin circles of white matter, formed by the fibro-vascular vessels; these circles can be easily separated by a longitudinal section in the dry root. The microscopical examination of the powdered root, or of a thin portion of it, presents a large number of crystals in the form of very fine needles set in small bundles. It can be observed also that no cribble vessels are apparent, as in the case of the *Chichicamole* root for which it has been, in some cases, mistaken on account of the great general resemblance.

The leaves of this plant are ovate-lanceolate, thin, obtusely-crenate, with very small points on the surface. The main vein is thick and projecting on the inferior surface.

The blossoms are set in bunches with small peduncles. They are of a white color, small, with eight stamens as long as the calyx and with persistent pistils.

Fruit. This is a purple colored berry as large as a common chick-pea, the seeds being lenticular and small. It flowering season is during the months of May and June.

CHEMICAL COMPOSITION—Has not been well established until now. We can only state that it was not found to contain any phytolacin nor any phytolacic acid.

PHYSIOLOGICAL ACTION—The fresh root has effective vomi-purgative properties. The dose that produced the most remarkable effects on small dogs, was that of 2 grammes by kilo of animal. No toxic effects were observed, neither with this dose nor with stronger ones. The dried root is not so active as the fresh one.

The fresh fruits have an emetic action. This effect is produced in small dogs with the dose of one gramme of the juice to kilo of animal.

THERAPEUTICAL EXPERIMENTS—The purgative effects of the fruit of Congora have not been established by the therapeutical experiments made at the Hospital of San Andrés, where it was employed in doses of one gramme of the fluid extract of the fruit.

Yerba del tabardillo.

SCIENTIFIC SYN—Piqueria trinervia, Cav. Ageratum febrifugum, Sesé et Mociño. Stevia fefrifuga, Sesé et Mociño ex D. C.

VULGAR SYN—Yoloxiltic, Xoxonitztac, or Xoxonitzal, Yerba de San Nicolas.

PLACES OF VEGETATION—It is very common in the Mexican Valley and in many other parts of the Republic.

PARTS EMPLOYED—The entire plant.

GENERAL CHARACTERS—Herbaceous, about one meter in height, the stem stout and sometimes pubescent and with two red lines extending its whole length. The branches are opposite; the leaves ovate-lanceolate, opposite, serrate, with three veins and glabrous surface. The inflorescence is in paniculate corymbs, with axilary and terminal peduncles; the capitulum is homogamus, tubuliform, 4 bracted, connivent, ovate, and membranous at the apex.

Its flowering season is during the months of August and September.

CHEMICAL COMPOSITION—

> Fat, in small proportion.
> Essential oil.
> Tannic acid.
> Resin.
> Extractive matter.
> Gum.
> Alkaloid (Piquerin).
> Alumin.
> Lime.
> Muriatic acid.

> —*F. Rio de la Loza, Inst. Med. Nac.* 1894.

The *Piquerin* is white, it is crystallized in prismatic needls, and has a slightly bitter taste; odorless, insoluble in the water, soluble in alcohol in the proportion of 0.30%. It is but slightly soluble in sulphuric ether, less in petroleum ether and still less in chloroform.

PHYSIOLOGICAL EXPERIMENTS—From several experiments that have been made at the Institute, we can state that the "Yerba del tabardillo" produces a decrease from the normal temperature.

THERAPEUTICAL EXPERIMENTS—It has been employed against intermittent fever and also against typhus, and it was observed that it acts in a similar manner to the *Contrayerba* and the antipyrin and that it can be considered as an antithermic.

DOSES AKD PREPARATIONS—Fluid extract of Piqueria 100 grammes in the 24 hours.

Capulincillo.

This drug, which grows in great abundance in the states of Queretaro, Hidalgo, Michoacan, etc., is nothing but a Rhamne, the Rhamnus Humboltianus (Rœmet, Schultz.)

It is a violent poison which produces paralysis. It is analogous in its physiological action to curare.

The fruits contain an oil which is neither toxic nor drying, and has no special odor or taste.

This drug has been employed, but with very little success, against hydrophobia and spasms.

Yoloxochitl.

Scientific Syn—Talauma mexicana, Magnolia grandiflora, Moc et Sessé, ex D. C.—M. glauca, Moc. et Sessé ex D. C.—M. mexicana, D. C.

Vulgar Syn—Flor del corazon, (Flower of the heart), Magnolia.

Habitat—It is found in the states of Morelos and Vera Cruz.

Parts Employed—Flowers, fruit and bark.

Characters of the Drug—The floral buttons are from 8 to 10 centimetres in length, ovate, cordiform, with numerous petals, white and fleshy in the fresh flowers and friable and of a yellowish brown color in the dry ones; the external petals are pubescent at the base of their external faces, the others are glabrous. They have a peculiar aromatic odor which is not observed in the dry ones.

Chemical Composition—Of the seed.

Fat, in the proportion of 56%.
Acid resin.
Neuter resin.
Essential oil.
Dyeing matter.
Extractive bitter matter.
Talaumin.
Resinous glucoside.
Salts of potasse and soda.
Oxalic acid.
Malic acid.
Iron.

—*Dr. Armendariz, Inst. Med. Nac.* 1894.

The *Talaumin* is a liquid of a red color. It has a bitter taste and forms crystallized salts which are soluble in water and in alcohol at 85°. It is but slightly soluble in ether, benzine and chloroform. The aqueous solutions of talaumin are decomposed by heat.

Physiological Action—The *Talaumin,* and above all the sulphate of talaumin, causes paralysis of the voluntary muscular system; the heart muscles are not affected by these symptoms. The glucoside of the talauma mexicana is, on the contrary, a cardiac moderator which does not affect the voluntary movements.

A decoction of the bark acts in a similar way to digitalis, in retarding the cardiac contractions and augmenting their strength. The medicine is quickly accumulated in the system and gives to the urine a disagreeable odor.

Therapeutical Experiments—According to the experiments made by Dr. Terres, the yoloxochitl is a good regulator of the heart movements and might be used as a substitute for digitalis.

Doses and Preparations—As for this we can only advise its employment in the same manner in which Dr. Terres has used it during his experiments; five grammes of the bark of yoloxochitl in 140 grammes of water for a decoction to be taken in three portions during the day.

Cuauchichic.

SCIENTIFIC SYN—Garrya racemosa, Ramirez.

VULGAR SYN—Chichicuahuitl.

PLACES OF VEGETATION—It is found in the Mexican Valley and in some other regions of the Republic.

PARTS EMPLOYED—The bark.

CHARACTERS OF THE DRUG—It has a gray color with whitish points on its surface, the size of the bark varying according to the size of the branch from which it has been obtained, it appears with its margins rolled inward, the external surface rugose, rough and scaly, the interior one is smooth and of a lighter color than the external one.

CHEMICAL COMPOSITION—

> Crystallizable bitter principle.
> Resin.
> Tannic acid.
> Extractive and gummy matters.

The active principle of the *Cuauchichic* was obtained by Dr. Armendaris who called it *Garrin.* It is a solid, crystallizable matter, fusible but not volatile, almost odorless, with a strong, bitter taste, very soluble in water and in alcohol. Nitric acid gives to it a pink color.

PHYSIOLOGICAL ACTION—From the experiments made at the institute with a decoction of the bark we can state:

First. That it is an active substance.

Second. That it causes death to rabbits when injected into those animals in doses above 8 c.c.

Third. That when the same decoction is employed in doses not larger than 5 c.c. it only produces an augmentation in the number and the extent of the respiratory movements. These symptoms pass away after a little time.

THERAPEUTICAL EXPERIMENTS—It has not been so employed until recently, but in cases of chronic diarrhœa we have found it to be very useful.

DOSES AND PREPARATIONS—Alcoholic tincture of Cuauchichic, three teaspoonfuls in a day.

Croton Morifolius,

Var Sphaerocarpus. (Euphorbaceous.)

SCIENTIFIC SYN—

VULGAR SYN—Palillo.

GROWS—In Guanajuato in dry and rough situations, where it is scarce if abundant rains do not fall.

PARTS EMPLOYED—The leaves and flowering summits.

GENERAL CHARACTERS—The leaves are elipsoidal, acuminate, tapering at the base, entire and tomentose on both surfaces but principally on the inferior one, this last character makes the leaf present a green color on the upper surface and a whitish on the inferior one. It is feather veined, with two strong ramifications that start at the same point from the base. The limb is very soft, flexible, aromatic, agreeable to taste and without causing any acridity on pharynx (this is an especial character which makes it differ from the Croton ciliato glandulosus for which it can be mistaken.) The inflorescence bears at the same time flowers and fruit with seeds more or less ripe. The flowers, are of a wool-white color, due to their being so tomentose. The fruits are of the size of a large chick-pea; they also are tomentose and this character gives them a yellowish color. Each fruit contains three seeds that resemble in form those of Ricinus. They have a shining surface with small brown spots. This drug can be obtained in large quantities at Guanajuato at the price of 4c a kilo. It is sold together with the stems which are hard, woody, and of no use.

CHEMICAL COMPOSITION—Essential oil, concrete fat, wax resin, yellow dyeing matter, a special tannic acid, glucoside, malic, citric and oxalic acids, a special acid, gummy, sugary and albuminous matters, and various salts.

The essential oil is the most important principle. It is liquid, very fluid and volatile (boiling point 33 C. G.), yellowish, with an agreeable, aromatic, strong and characteristic smell, which resembles that of the fresh plant. It has a burning resinous taste, is lighter than water in which it is but slightly soluble, though soluble in alcohol. It appears mixed with some other essential oils in which the boiling point is from 120 to 150 C. G. It oxydizes in contact with the air and it is probable that it contains oxygen in its elemental composition.

The glucoside is solid, yellowish, non-crystallizable, without any odor and of a slightly bitter taste; it is soluble in the water and also in alcohol and gives, with the proper agents, the different reactions, characteristic of the glucosides.

PHYSIOLOGIC ACTION—The active principle of this herb is the essential oil. It acts upon the nervous system, diminishing its excitability by peripheric and central action. It causes local anæsthesia when it is used *loco dolente*. When inhaled, it causes insensibility and paralysis of movement. When it is ingested, it causes local anæsthesia of the stomach. The decoction made with the ground inflorescence causes purgative effects which are due, perhaps, to the seeds. The sub-cutaneous injection of two or four drops of the essence causes stupefaction and cerebral depression in the frog one minute after the injection, and later, loss of muscular energy, and general paresis, suspension of the respiratory movements but not of the cardiac ones; diminution of the cutaneous and corneous reflex; conservation of the muscular exitability and of the motor and sensitive nerves at their extremities. Two hours later these symptoms disappear, and the animal recovers its normal state. So that the absorption and the elimination of this medicine takes place with great rapidity. By following the method of Bernard, it has been demonstrated that this essence causes anæsthesia of the cutaneous surfaces and that of the nerves of sensation. This effect was produced with the infusion, with the tincture and with the essence, but it was not obtained with the liquid taken after a long decoction.

THERAPEUTICAL EXPERIMENTS—The physicians have employed it successfully during their town-practice and at the hospital against facial neuralgia and gastralgies. The tincture is used for relieving pain. It acts best when it operates directly upon the extremities of the sensitive nerves.

POSOLOGY—The fluid extract is given internally at doses of 2 to 4 grammes a day; the tincture from 10 to 15 grammes, in several doses during the day; the essential oil in doses of 1 to 4 drops in an alcoholic or olive oil solution put in gelatine capsules; the tea-form infusion in the proportion of 10 to 15%. For external use the tincture is used by applying it with friction *loco dolente*.

Helenium Mexicanum, H. B. K.

(Compositæ.)

Scientific Syn—Helenium integrifolium, Moc. and Sessé, Fl. Mex.

Vulgar Syn—Chapuz, Herb of the Ghosts, Rosilla, Cabezona.

Grows—In the Mexican Valley, Morelia, Queretaro and Guanajuato. It generally vegetates in wet and marshy lands, where it is found growing in compact masses. Its flowering season is during the months of July and August till November.

Parts Employed—The capitulum or flower head. These are sold more or less ground. They can be obtained in large quantities in Mexico at the price of $0.50c a kilo.

Characters of the Capitulum—Almost spherical, brown colored, from 1 to 2 centimetres in diameter, bearing dry, furrowed and yellow colored bracts at the base. The black color is due to a dyeing matter which exists in the papillæ that are on the external surface of the corolla. The receptacle is conoid, slightly alveolate, and the interior is hollowed and generally full of insects. It has an aromatic odor which resembles in some degree that of chamomilla. When the powder gets into the nose, though in small quantities, it causes violent and persistent sneezing.

Chemical Composition—Concrete oil, acid resin, essential oil, yellow dyeing matter, alkaloid, tannic acid, tartaric acid, albumen, gum and mineral salts. The resin and the alkaloid are the active principles of this plant. (See "Datos para la Materia Médica Mexicana.") The alkaloid has a bitter and pungent taste. It is little soluble in water, but entirely soluble in alcohol, ether and chloroform. It is easily combined with the acids and forms with them crystallizable salts.

Physiologic Action—The resin is an energetic irritant, and it is to this action that the errhinic effects are chiefly due. It acts in the intestines as a powerful and dangerous drastic.

The absorption of the alkaloid when applied by subcutaneous injection, is very rapid, the first symptoms having appeared, in some cases, within a few seconds. Twenty or thirty minutes later, the symptoms become very intense and death occurs after one or two hours, according to the dose employed. The most remarkable symptoms that have been observed in the rabbit, in the frog and in the dog are general epileptic convulsions, alternate with paralysis of the motility, myosis, midriasis, ptosis, salivation, and mastication movements. The convulsions cease a short time before death, succeeded by a general flaccidity and death, at last, generally occurs by the paralysis of the respiration, within one or two hours, according to the dose employed.

THERAPEUTICAL EXPERIMENTS—The Chapuz has been employed at the Hospital of San Andrés, obtaining in every case different results. It was employed against locomotor ataxia and proved useful in calming the pains, and in some cases it rendered the patients able to walk. It was employed also against epilepsy, but without obtaining any favorable effects.

People make use of the chapuz against chronic catarrh and also to establish the prognostic in serious cases of typhus. In the last case they introduce into the patient's nose a small quantity of powdered chapuz, and if the patient sneezes, he will recover, otherwise death is certain. The people in the country use the chapuz to kill the worms that in some instances invade the wounds of the animals. To apply the drug they make a paste, mixing the chapuz, previously ground, with powdered lime, then they apply this paste to the wounds, killing the worms. It is said, too, that the powdered flowers are useful for exterminating the head louse and may be used in place of cebadilla (Veratrum cebadilla.) It can be deduced from all this that the chapuz is a good insecticide, though very dangerous to man.

POSOLOGY—The posology of this plant is not yet well determined. The powder of the flowers has been given to patients at the hospital, beginning with doses of one miligram, until it reached one centigramme in 24 hours. In one case the dose was raised to 1 gramme and 30 centigrammes.

The resin has been experimented with in doses of 2 grammes, causing the animal's death.

The alkaloid has not been entirely isolated till now, and for this reason the dose of it has not been fixed.

Comino.

(Cumin, Eng.)

SCIENTIFIC SYN—Cuminum cyminum, L.

PLACES OF VEGETATION—In the High Nile. It is cultivated in Mexico.

PARTS EMPLOYED—The fruit.

CHEMICAL COMPOSITION—

> Essential oil.
> Resin.
> Fat oil.
> Mucilage, etc.

ECONOMICAL USES—As a condiment.

MEDICINAL USES—Stimulant and carminative.

Cominos rusticos.

SCIENTIFIC SYN—Aracacia multifida, Wats.

PLACES OF VEGETATION—It grows in the Mexican Valley.

PARTS EMPLOYED—The fruit.

CHARACTERS OF THE FRUIT—Oblong-elliptical, compressed on one side; the mericarp has five sides, three dorsal ones and two larger marginal ones. They have an aromatic acid flavor and their odor resembles that of fennel.

CHEMICAL COMPOSITION—It contains a large quantity of essential oil which has been extracted at the Institute.

USES—It is commonly employed as a stimulant and anti-blenorrhagic.

Cacahuananche.

SCIENTIFIC SYN—Licania arborea, Seem.

VULGAR SYN—Quirindal.

PLACES OF VEGETATION—In the states of Guerrero, Morelos and Michoacan.

GENERAL CHARACTERS—The seeds have the form and dimension of an olive fruit. They are of a light coffee color and have a persistent disagreeable, rancid odor. They ignite easily in contact with flame and continue burning by themselves on account of the large proportion of oil that they contain. They have two plano-convex cotyledons, which are fleshy and become hard by dessication.

The oil obtained from the Cacahuananche can be easily saponified into a very hard soap. It contains a grease acid, very solid and fusible at 88°. This could be employed in the manufacture of bougies (candles.)

Cascalote.

SCIENTIFIC SYN—Cœsalpina cacalaco, H. B. K.

PLACES OF VEGETATION—Michoacan, Guerrero and Oaxaca.

The fruit is the part of this plant employed in economics. It contains a large quantity of tannic acid and a small proportion of dyeing matter, and is used for tanning the skins of animals.

Tabaquillo.

SCIENTIFIC SYN—Calamintha macrostema.

VULGAR SYN—Tea of the mountain, Tabaquillo tea.

PLACES OF VEGETATION—In the mountains of the Mexican Valley and in many other places of the Republic.

PARTS EMPLOYED—The leaves.

GENERAL CHARACTERS OF THE PLANT—Shrub, the stems are lignious, four-angled, and of a brown color; the leaves are simple, opposite, thin, ovate-lanceolate, from 3 to 6 centimetres in length and from 1 to 1½ in width, dentate, velvety and with numerous glands which can be easily observed on the inferior surface; the petioles are from 10 to 14 milimetres in length. The leaves are very aromatic and with an agreeable taste.

CHEMICAL COMPOSITION—The analysis of this plant is not yet finished. We have only obtained the essential oil by distillation of the plant, it contains a large quantity of it and can be employed as that of the Mentha piperita.

PHYSIOLOGICAL ACTION—A diluted solution of the essence was employed for these experiments, and it was found that it causes the anæsthesia in the extremities of the sensitive nerves. It provokes symptoms of narcotism, when it is employed in large doses.

THERAPEUTICAL EXPERIMENTS—We can state from several experiments that have been made, that it has been successfully employed to ease the pains of gastralgia and for stimulating the intestinal movements. It could be employed as a good stomachic in a tea-form infusion.

DOSES AND PREPARATIONS—Aqueous infusion of the leaves of Tabaquillo, from 5 to 10%—100 grammes.
Alcoholic tincture—from 40 to 50 drops.

Altamisa or Artemisa del país.

SCIENTIFIC SYN—Ambrosia artemisiæfolia, L.
PLACES OF VEGETATION—It is found in abundance in the Mexican Valley.

CHARACTERS—It is characterized by its capitulums which are inverted and set in terminal spikes; the leaves are pinnate-lobed, the lobes are pinnatifid, amplexicual and rough, they have numerous hairs on their surface. Their aromatic odor resembles in much that of absinthium, they have a sour bitter taste.

The most important principles that it contains are the essential oil, resin and tannic acid.

Made in the USA
Las Vegas, NV
16 December 2024

e66b19f2-d26b-4b54-9fb3-038c228d786dR01